Improving Services for Older People

Staff development in dementia care

Mary Fraser
Director, Research & Project Consultancy, Stirling

Stanley Thornes (Publishers) Ltd

First published in 1999 by:
Stanley Thornes (Publishers) Ltd
Ellenborough House
Wellington Street
Cheltenham
Glos.
GL50 1YW
United Kingdom

99 00 01 02 03 / 10 9 8 7 6 5 4 3 2 1

A catalogue record for this book is available from the British Library

ISBN 0 7487 3896 7

Typeset by Acorn Bookwork, Salisbury, Wiltshire
Printed and bound in Great Britain by TJ International Ltd, Padstow, Cornwall

CONTENTS

PREFACE

This book is about learning how to care for people with dementia, where carers are either paid employees or volunteers. It assumes that carers undertake this kind of work because they enjoy it. It also assumes that everyone is capable, provided they are motivated enough, to learn from the experiences that they enjoy. Therefore, care for people with dementia seems like an ideal situation in which learning by working can become a reality.

In this book I begin by considering the context in which care for older people is being carried out at the end of the 20th century in the UK. It is undoubtedly fraught with problems, not least of which is funding and finance. However, despite much of the care being in the private sector, which must make a profit in order to stay in business, the quality of care is variable and is seen to be in need of regulation. It is against this background that continuing to improve the quality of care is set. If the willingness to work with people with dementia is harnessed by the organisation and the carers are encouraged to learn as they work, the potential for continued improvement could be realised.

In Chapter 1 I consider the national trends in population and care for older people, particularly in the private and voluntary sectors, as this is where the majority of old people in care are being cared for. Chapter 2 considers the ways in which high-quality care is currently being developed along the lines of quality of life while adhering to ideas of best value. Both these notions are developed for the people with dementia as well as for the carers and managers. Chapter 3 discusses various forms of training, as training is now very important in care and it is no longer expected that carers will have natural aptitudes for caring without any training for the work. Notions of life-long learning are developed and their appropriateness suggested for these types of organisations.

In Chapter 4 I begin to consider how life-long learning can be analysed and made a reality in care for people with dementia. By working with carers, helping them to discuss problems and possible solutions, I develop a way of introducing notions of learning from experience to produce change. Chapters 5 and 6 give detail of the structure of teaching and working with eight very different organisations that care for a variety of people with dementia. Using the contents of Chapters 4 and 5, I discuss the organisations' individual reactions to self-directed learning, the impact of such an attempt on the senior carers and the organisations with whom I worked, and the potential for the people with dementia.

In the last chapter I have made a few suggestions as to how self-directed life-long learning can become a reality in care for older people with dementia and also how this reflects on the organisations with whom I had contact.

I am most grateful to the organisations with whom I worked. I feel they are undertaking an immensely necessary role in very difficult circumstances. I hope that they will take the conclusions I have made in the spirit of trying to be helpful and will consider that I have made a useful contribution to their efforts. I wish them all well.

My thanks also go, as ever, to my husband Sandy. Without his continual encouragement and support this book would not have materialised.

Mary Fraser
Director
Research & Project Consultancy
Tower Orchard House
Cambuskenneth
STIRLING
FK9 5NH
Tel/Fax: 01786 450824
E-mail: 101326.3306@compuserve.com

1 INTRODUCTION: THE CONTEXT OF CARE FOR OLDER PEOPLE IN THE UK

This book is about the growing need for care for people with dementia in the UK. It highlights the context in which this care is given, mainly in the private and voluntary sectors. It also considers one of the most pressing needs – that of the continual striving for improved quality. That is not to say that quality is necessarily poor – far from it – but as each organisation caring for people with dementia comes under increasing scrutiny from a whole variety of bodies, the need to demonstrate quality becomes more pressing.

This chapter introduces care for older people in the community in the UK. As long-term care is now barely recognised as part of the National Health Service, I look at the kinds of services that are available but, more importantly, put these in the context of either private sector care, in which profit is essential to staying in business, or voluntary sector care, in which charitable status is important for funding. But, whether private or voluntary, care for older people has to take place within certain principles which are usually associated with good business practice, such as identifying who your clients are, knowing what their needs are and gearing your services to their needs while being competitive and having an eye on what your competitors are offering.

According to Barrow & Brown (1997), once a business has survived the initial years of setting up, the next stage is the challenge of staying in business. The main difficulties at this stage can be summed up as:

- Determining the key factors for success in your business sector.
- Developing a balanced management team.
- Further developing your market differentiation.
- Funding future growth. (p. 83)

Those who are not operating on these principles are, according to Barrow & Brown, unlikely to stay in business for any length of time. They emphasise the point, by showing the sharp increase in the possibility of going into liquidation depending on the age of the business. It would seem that after 30 months there is a sharp increase in businesses ceasing to trade, with one-third of small firms going out of business in the first three years. The chance of success does not improve with length of time, as within the first 10 years nearly two-thirds of those who initially set up will not survive. It should be noted that Barrow & Brown are particularly referring to small businesses; however, many nursing and residential homes and community organisations, even those in a large chain, operate as small businesses, so their point is well made. They are also speaking about all types of small business; however, care cannot be divorced from this trend and there is evidence that homes for older people are just as likely to go out of business as any other type of enterprise. Evidence of survival rates is given by Judy Hirst in *Community Care* in October, 1997, when discussing decreasing bed occupancy rates in nursing and residential homes, from over 90% in the early 1990s to around 85% in 1997 (see also Laing & Buisson, 1997). Evidence is also provided by one chain of nursing homes that has developed a service for homes that cease to trade while still having residents and staff to be considered. Judy Hirst suggests that developing into 'niche' markets may be a solution to lower bed occupancy. Laing & Buisson agree and also point to the development of psychiatric services.

Therefore, in this context, let us look at a number of factors, such as who your clients are, what they need from the service and what it costs as well as how this has changed within the last 15 years, the competition in the care sector and the constraints under which each organisation operates. This will cover at least three of Barrow & Brown's criteria for staying in business, namely 'the key factors for success in your business sector'; 'developing your market differentiation' and 'funding future growth'. This will form the contents of this chapter.

WHO ARE YOUR CLIENTS? THE DEMOGRAPHICS OF OLDER AGE

Although most people know about the increasing age of the population, no book on care for older people can really be complete without a brief mention of this. I therefore intend to give a few statistics about the increasing age of people in the UK and what we might expect in the next few years.

According to *Population Trends*, the government statistical publication, the number of men and women in the UK of pensionable age is set to increase from 10.6 million in 1992 to 11.9 million in 2010. A further increase to 15.2 million is projected to occur up to the year 2038. Due to improvements in medicine, the numbers who survive into very old age, usually defined as over 75 years, are also likely to be considerable. Of those of pensionable age, the over-75 age group are the most likely to develop dementia, therefore are more likely to need the most care. In 1987 it was estimated that one in three residents in care had dementia (Hunter, 1987). Of those who do not develop dementia, living alone is most likely to result in poor health and increasing frailty (McGarrity & Knox, 1995). Therefore, because of the longer life expectancy of women, they can expect to be more likely to live alone in their older age.

Laing & Buisson (1997) estimate there will be an increase in the numbers of people over 85 years until the year 2001 and then a dip will occur between the years 2001 and 2004 due to the decline in the birth rate during the First World War years. From 2005 the upward trend will continue. However, according to the Royal Commission (Sutherland, 1999), this does not constitute a 'demographic time-bomb', as has been feared by some and has been widely discussed. They say therefore that 'the costs of care will be affordable' (p. xviii) in the UK.

WHAT DO THE CLIENTS NEED FROM THE SERVICE AND WHAT DOES IT COST?

There has been increasing encouragement from government for public and private sector health care to work together; this has been since at least the beginning of the 1980s (see DHSS circular HC(81)1) when a form of deregulation was introduced. There was also the expectation that the private sector would grow and was to be encouraged. This indicated the changes in regulation introduced in the Acts of 1984 (Registered Homes Act, 1984; The Residential Care Homes Regulations, 1984).

The years surrounding the new Acts saw much debate about care for older people, at this time more often in an institution rather than in the person's own home. Debate centred around three main themes.

First, that residents were increasingly frail. This was causing a particular problem in residential homes where many reports showed the number of areas of dependency of some residents, which included inability to wash unaided; severe confusion; double incontinence; inability to feed themselves; and non-mobility (see Armstrong, 1984). Therefore the distinction between older people in residential and nursing homes was becoming increasingly blurred.

The trend of increasing dependency among residents in nursing and residential homes has increased. According to the Independent Health Care Association in 1997, the results of their national survey of 320 homes showed that dependency scores had risen by 27% since 1993.

Second, that the increasing dependency of residents was causing pressure on community services, such as GPs and district nurses. Whereas GPs were responsible for residents' medical care, a lack of training of care staff led to their inability to recognise and treat problems of increasing age and infirmity. This was combined with information and advice about services that could be provided failing to reach the homes. By the end of 1995 it was evident that the numbers of older people being cared for in long-term NHS beds had declined considerably and the majority of care was being undertaken outside the NHS (Harding, 1995).

This transfer of care for older people into the community with the resulting pressures on services reached crisis point at the end of 1996, with the British Medical Association (BMA) saying that consultations in nursing and residential homes were 10 times more than the national average. As residents were increasingly frail and bedridden, GPs could no longer treat them as one of their 'core' services; doctors could decide whether or not to offer their services (see Hirst, 1996). This move was intended to protect the essence of general practice from becoming submerged by the needs of residents, to the detriment of the GPs' quality of care.

Third, the methods of paying for care lacked cohesion (some people were privately funded, some funded by health authorities, some by supplementary benefits) and costs escalated rapidly. In autumn 1983 the DHSS undertook a tidying up exercise which asked supplementary benefits offices to fix a schedule of maximum fees for older people in private and voluntary care, which should depend on local charges. This meant that older people who did not have the financial means to pay for their care could be admitted to and kept in private and voluntary homes, almost on demand. Whereas admission to private and voluntary care from the NHS was assessed by health professionals using professional criteria, the supplementary benefits offices took only financial need into account. The limits fixed by benefits offices were well in excess of previous rates and were not cash limited; Challis, Day & Klein (1984) show rises of over 400% from £55 per week to £200 for residential homes and £300 per week for nursing homes in one London borough. These levels of increase were repeated around the UK, whereas domiciliary services, such as meals on wheels, were not supported. Therefore most private and voluntary homes put up their prices to the maximum limit. Due to the increases and lack of co-ordination between government departments, the discharge of older people from hospital into long-stay care became too expensive, as health authorities were not geared up to such rates, and therefore, large-scale bed blocking occurred. The scandal this caused was noted in *The Sunday Times* in October 1984.

The increase in benefits along with encouragement from banks to take out loans to set up private nursing and residential care led to one of the largest increases in private sector care for older people that the UK had known. In 1987 funding for older people in private care from the public purse stood at around £500m and was forecast to rise dramatically. However, the number of inspectors of homes did not match this so there was real concern for the quality of care. By 1994, the first year of the Community Care Act being in operation, spending in England alone was £874 million (Department of Health, 1996). Since the Community Care Act, a similar increase was noted in services outside full residential care, such as day centres, meals, home helps and adaptations to houses. Whereas in 1986 spending was £348 million, by 1993–4 this had risen to £779 million, an increase in real terms of 49% (Department of Health, 1996).

In 1987, a DHSS working party recommended that responsibility for all residential care should be passed to local government but recognised the rift and interprofessional rivalry between health and social services (Hunter, 1987). When this notion was developed into the Community Care Act, operational since 1993, responsibility for care of older people outside hospital became the province of social services departments within councils. Therefore, from this moment on, local government became the managers of local services, rather than the providers. To allow for transitional arrangements, special transitional grants were made available which were gradually incorporated into social services budgets. From this time, with continual constraints on public spending and particularly on councils' budgets, claims of funding crises became more prevalent. While many social services departments overspent their budgets in 1995–6, this resulted in having to make savings in 1996–7 to compensate.

While there have always been services for those who can pay for them, challenges to providing services from public funds saw test cases in the High Court, such as those brought against Gloucestershire County Council and the London Borough of Islington (see Dobson, 1995). In these cases the law confirmed that social services cannot simply withdraw services once they have been agreed and provided without a reassessment of the individual's needs. However, services did not have to be provided initially if there were not the resources to pay for them; this then could open the way for those needing services to have to pay for them. Assessments of need from this point led to increasing waiting lists for services and claims that they were not needs led but resources led, which threatened the emphasis on choice of services by the individual needing them, one of the main aims of community care (see O'Kell, 1996). From at least 1995 charges for public sector services were made which were almost bound to increase annually, although services were not always able to be provided to those who needed them (Baldwin & Lunt, 1996). In 1996 it was expected that 10% of the cost of services would be met by charging (Neate, 1996). It was also unknown how many people were not using services due to the cost.

With the expansion of services to people in their own homes, expansion of the domiciliary sector seemed inevitable as a result of community care. However, by 1995 there seemed to be little evidence of such expansion in the private sector (Young & Wistow, 1995). This was felt to be mainly due to inconsistent support from local authorities which led to there being few incentives for providers when funding might be withdrawn as budgetary pressures increase (Policy Studies Institute, 1996).

Voluntary services, such as Crossroads care attendant scheme, also showed a considerable increase in their workload but with decreased budgets (see CNA report, 1997). In fact, the Policy Studies Institute (1996) found that sustaining services was a problem and many voluntary services ceased to operate during the period 1992–5, while others folded shortly afterwards. As the voluntary sector also relies in large part on contracting with local government (National Commission on the Future of the Voluntary Sector, 1996) this means that as the financial uncertainty in local government increases, so the uncertainty of service provision in the voluntary sector also increases. However, by 1996, 18 schemes around the UK to ease the discharge of older people from hospitals had been agreed between social services departments, health authorities and health trusts (Henwood & Waddington, 1996; Carlisle, 1996).

In May 1996 the government's mixed economy of welfare policies (the combination of public, private, voluntary and informal sector care) saw another turn with John Major's announcement of insurance schemes to cover long-term care. This led certain insurance companies to develop policies and, increasingly, accountants and lawyers to became involved in issues pertaining to older people's care. However, whereas most insurance companies and accountants were solely interested in financial planning for old age, lawyers were also concerned with the quality of the care that could be provided with the finances.

Further recent developments in care in the domestic setting have involved schemes for direct payments to those needing care which, following an assessment by social workers, reflects the level of funding needed to provide that care. Therefore the person needing care has responsibility to provide their own care from the direct payment. How this will work is currently being debated and scrutinised using pilot studies in various parts of the country. However, according to the King's Fund, help in achieving alterations to houses to assist older people to stay at home is also not being adequately funded (BBC Radio 4, 1998).

Summarising the needs of clients and the costs of services, it would appear that despite the large increase in the cost of care to the public purse since the mid 1980s, as well as the beginnings of charging for services, there is likely to be a large pool of unmet need, particularly from those less able to pay. This reflects the inequalities in society which have become more evident over the last two decades and which the Joseph Rowntree report highlighted in 1995. With the change in government in May 1997 a Royal Commission was set up, under the chairmanship of Sir Stewart Sutherland, to consider options for a sustainable system of funding for long-term care. The Commission recommended that provision should be shared between the individual and the state, where state resources should be fair, equitable and transparent. The whole area of long-term care is currently very dynamic, as Tony Blair has consistently indicated his wish to see reforms of the welfare state.

WHAT IS THE COMPETITION IN THE CARE SECTOR?

Despite the picture painted in the previous section, can we assume that once an older person receives services their needs are met? Competition in the private care sector is fierce; therefore this section deals with competition in the sector in order to stay in business.

To keep the beds or the day centre places full is vital to success or else revenue falls. However, competitive prices are only one aspect as quality of care and reputation are vital as well as the type of accommodation and services offered. Apart from clients who pay privately for services, since the Community Care Act, social services have seen their role as managing the placements of older people according to the latter's wishes and the places available. Therefore, for a private organisation, approval by registration and inspection services is essential to achieving referrals paid for from the public purse. Although there have been numerous calls from the private sector for self-regulation (see, for example, *Community Care*, 1995), this is still firmly in the hands of local authority and health authority registration and inspection units. However, this is a very contentious issue as homes and services provided by the local authority do not have to undergo inspection. It is also an anomaly that the local authority can act as regulator and provider, a fact that private owners are not slow to point out when their occupancy rates fall! In recent years, however, the number of local authority services for older people have fallen, with the closure or selling off of homes, leaving the private sector with the majority of services in most parts of the UK. But the place of registration and inspection units and their affiliations is a persistent issue with continuing calls for inspection to be separated from provision of services (see Valios, 1997). There is also recent evidence that Registration and Inspection units have merged as joint inspection units (see *Community Care*, 1997), so the emphasis of community care on joint professional working between health and social services is starting to be seen more clearly.

Inspection of private facilities takes place at least twice a year and formal reports are made to the homes with recommendations of where improvements are needed. These are public documents, so homes are very keen to be seen in the best light possible. However, the standards by which services for older people are inspected have also been the subject of fierce debate over a period of years. In line with Donabedian's (1966) criteria of structure, process and outcome, the structure of the building and the physical facilities have been the most tangible evidence of service quality. Therefore, recent debates about shared rooms for residents have led to many existing homes converting or building new extensions with single en-suite facilities. Structure also includes adherence to health and safety legislation, fire precautions, safe storage of dangerous chemicals and policies on food preparation, storage and disposal. As well as health and safety legislation, there is also legislation on the storage of medicines.

However, it is the process and outcome part of Donabedian's criteria which has been the most difficult to measure and the subject of numerous reports and guides to standards (see, for example, Residential Forum, 1996; Centre for Policy on Ageing, 1996). The most enduring current theme is providing quality of life for older people including giving choice in the services and their provision. This will not be further developed here as it could be the subject of an entire book in itself; however, quality of life as a theme will be covered in later chapters when we consider staff training in detail.

A further recurrent theme has been training for inspectors which arises whenever issues of abuse reach the headlines. The National Association of Registration and Inspection Officers has been calling for a national training programme and a formal qualification for officers (see Valios, 1997) for a number of years. However, although vocational qualifications for officers exist, they do not seem to be well supported (Laming, 1996–7).

As part of ensuring standards in the process of care, vocational qualifications (VQs) now play a large part in private sector care and staff training to a recognised level is starting to form part of contract specifications (George, 1997). Recognised training is important as the care sector mainly recruits women with no formal education and who often have left school with few qualifications; the work can also be notoriously badly paid (Platt, 1997). So organisations that can show they have some of their staff trained to VQ level will have an advantage. However, as George indicates, funding for such training is seldom available from the local authorities. There are also large variations in local training and enterprise council awards towards funding VQs.

The take-up of VQs has been good in the private and voluntary sectors, but they have been less well taken up in the public sector (George, 1997). Also some organisations prefer to send their staff on courses or run in-house training, although the standards of the latter can be variable.

While training for carers has become well recognised, training for managers has also been subject to scrutiny. New managers are being expected not only to posses experience in the sector but increasingly to hold management qualifications, either at VQ level III or IV or HND, or to have undertaken business courses supported by the enterprise companies, such as Investors in People. The latter have made a significant impact in England.

Summarising competition in care, it would be fair to say that a good report by the inspection team is one of the most important issues to providers of services. This guides their developments and they rely heavily on information given by inspectors for the further development of services. Therefore the management of services for older people in the community by social services is starting to be seen more clearly. However, it would be true to say that inspectors themselves are undergoing a considerable period of transition due to the large increase in their workload with the expansion of private sector care. Along with this are the continuing debates about which organisation should be responsible for inspection services. The pressures on inspectors are, of course, raised when poor standards are uncovered and threats of withdrawal of registration loom.

SUMMARY

In this chapter we have looked at three main issues: the key factors to success in care for older people; developing your services and becoming competitive; and ways in which the organisation can grow. We have seen that although the number of older people and their needs for care continue to increase, the funding for this care has been a continuing and escalating problem. This is in part due to the welfare state which created the expectation that we would all be cared for in our old age without the expectation that we would have to provide for ourselves, which has now produced a reluctance to do so (Parker & Clarke, 1997). However, many Western nations with developed systems of welfare provision face a similar situation. Therefore, although there is no shortage of clients needing care, the ability of providers to achieve funding for the care they offer is the issue. To achieve full bed occupancy, one of the most important aspects is ensuring that increasing legal requirements are met and that one's reputation as a good organisation is maintained with the purchasers. There is also an increasing need to offer services which cater for particular sectors of the market, for example specialist dementia care, day services, respite care and psychiatric services. Ensuring recognised training is in place for care staff is a further major factor in the recognition of good quality as well as other forms of management training for owners and managers, such as Investors in People.

Despite problems of funding long-term care and the Royal Commission's recommendations, the number and size of private establishments have continued to increase. However, there is evidence that these are mainly the larger chains of homes who are able to consolidate in order to reduce administrative costs (Laing & Buisson, 1997). According to the Laing & Buisson study, mergers between these larger companies are increasingly likely, indicating fierce competition and also an increasing trend to provide services in European countries as well as in the UK.

In the next chapter we will be developing some of the areas discussed in this chapter further and focusing more on the delivery of care in nursing and residential homes and in community organisations. This will particularly be in relation to quality of care and cost effectiveness, including staff training and staff retention.

REFERENCES

Armstrong, J. (1984) Getting their act together. *Nursing Times*, 24 October, 38–40.
Baldwin, S. and Lunt, N. (1996) *Charging Ahead: Local Authority Charging*

Policies for Community Care. Joseph Rowntree Foundation and Polity Press, York.

Barrow, C. and Brown, R. (1997) *Principles of Small Business.* International Thomson Business Press, London.

BBC Radio 4 (1998) *Medicine Now,* 3rd February.

Carlisle, D. (1996) Quality time. *Community Care,* 22–28 August, 23.

Centre for Policy on Ageing (1996) *A Better Home Life.* CPA, London.

Challis, L., Day, P. and Klein, R. (1984) Residential care on demand. *New Society,* 5 April, 32.

CNA/ADSW/ADSS (1997) *In on the Act: Social Services' Experience of the First Year of the Carers Act.* Carers National Association, London.

Community Care (1995) Self-regulation favoured by home owners, not by users. 2–8 November, 3.

Community Care (1997) Scots establish first joint inspection unit. 24–30 July, 3.

Department of Health (1981*) Contractual Arrangements with Independent Hospitals and Nursing Homes and Other Forms of Co-operation Between the NHS and the Independent Medical Sector.* HC(81)1 HMSO, London.

Department of Health (1996) *Personal Social Services: A Historical Profile of Reported Current and Capital Expenditure 1983–84 to 1993–94.* HMSO, London.

Dobson, R. (1995) Death of an ideal, *Community Care,* 6–12 July, 8–9.

Donabedian, A. (1966) Evaluating the quality of medical care. *Milbank Memorial Fund Quarterly,* 64(3), part 2, 166–206.

George, M. (1997) Qualified to cope. *Community Care,* 17–23 April, 26–27.

Harding, T. (1995) Into the wilderness. *Community Care,* 27 April–3 May, 20–21.

Henwood, M. and Waddington, E. (1996) *Going Home: Report of an Evaluation of the British Red Cross Home from Hospital Initiative.* British Red Cross, London.

Hirst, J. (1996) Onto the scrap heap. *Community Care,* 28 November– 4 December, 10–11.

Hirst, J. (1997) This time it's personal. *Community Care,* 16–22 October, 26–27.

Hunter, D. (1987) Confused? You will be … *Health Service Journal,* 3 September, 1013.

Laing and Buisson (1997) *Care of Elderly People Market Survey,* Laing and Buisson Publications Ltd.

Laming, H. (1996–7) *Better Managed Better Care.* Social Services Inspectorate, London.

McGarrity, C. and Knox, B. (1995) Socio-economic determinants of dietary habits. *Social Sciences in Health,* 1(2), 94–106.

National Commission on the Future of the Voluntary Sector (1996) *Meeting the Challenges of Change: Voluntary Action into the 21st Century.* NCVO, London.

Neate, P. (1996) Strapped for cash. *Community Care,* 1–7 August, vi–viii.

O'Kell, S. (1996) Short changed, *Community Care*, 18–24 April, 26–27.

Parker, G. and Clarke, H. (1997) Will you still need me, will you still feed me? Paying for care in old age. *Social Policy and Administration*, 31(2), 119–135.

Platt, S. (1997) Qualifying rounds. *Community Care*, 30 January–5 February, 32–33.

Policy Studies Institute (1996) *Creating Partnerships in Social Care*. Grantham Books, Grantham.

Residential Forum (1996) *Creating a Home from Home*. Residential Forum, London.

Sunday Times (1984) Old at risk from DHSS blunder. p. 7.

Sutherland, S. (1999) *With Respect to Old Age: Long Term Care – Rights and Responsibilities*. A Report by the Royal Commission on Long Term Care. The Stationery Office, London.

Valios, N. (1997) Inspection abuse. *Community Care*, 17–23 July, 10–11.

Young, R. and Wistow, G. (1995) *Experiences of Independent Home Care Providers: Analysis of the January 1995 UKHCA Survey*. Nuffield Institute for Health, Oxford.

2 THE PROVISION OF HIGH-QUALITY CARE TO OLDER PEOPLE

In the last chapter we looked at the context in which care for older people is provided in the UK. We particularly concentrated on the patterns of care and the trends that have emerged, as well as the likely future prospects. We saw how maintaining a good reputation with the purchasers of care, largely using public money, was essential to staying in business as a private or voluntary care provider in a very dynamic field.

In this chapter we will develop this further and consider the basis on which the good reputation is maintained. There are a number of issues that play a part in this, therefore we will cover how high-quality care is defined by the public purchasers (social services). This will be linked to how cost effectiveness in purchasing and providing can be achieved and to staff training and staff retention. However, it is important to start by considering why high-quality care is important.

WHY IS HIGH-QUALITY CARE IMPORTANT?

Older people who need care are some of the most vulnerable in society. This is mainly because they are not only likely to be physically frail but in our culture, unlike some others, older people are not generally seen as having a great deal to contribute. We tend to value people who are economically active and independent; therefore, no matter what someone's previous position or role may have been, if they are no longer able to provide for themselves they become dependent on others, which lessens their value in our society (Bytheway, 1995). Those who are dependent are therefore more vulnerable, particularly if they have nobody to speak up for them. Quality of care is geared towards ensuring their vulnerability is not exploited by lack of knowledge, poor management or evil intent or a combination of all three.

WHAT IS HIGH-QUALITY CARE?

While we all have our own definitions of high-quality goods or services, in the context of care for older people purchased by the local authority it has a particular set of values. These are generally known as being within the remit of quality of life. The concept of quality of life has been developed in both the academic and professional settings to the extent that one eminent authority on the issue, Schalock, a Canadian social scientist, said in 1989 that it would be *the* issue in the human services in the 1990s.

Quality of life is difficult to define precisely. Seed & Lloyd (1997) say it is:

> *simultaneously about the needs and hopes of individual people and about groups of people. It is also about an individual's personal environment (the setting of their daily living).* (p. 4)

Therefore it encompasses almost every aspect of one's daily life. So, let us look at how this can be assessed in services to older people. What kinds of areas would be covered in providing good quality care?

From Figure 2.1 we can see there are a number of aspects. First, it assumes that those who provide the care and those who receive it fully understand the needs and hopes of each other. This is not only about providing care for older people, it also means that the conditions in which the carers work meet *their* needs and hopes as well (we will return to this later). Let us start by considering how the needs and hopes of older individuals can be known by their carers. This implies a great deal of sensitivity on the part of those who care for older people, not only to take every step to understand what they say and intend but also to be able to put this in the context of the older person's values. For example, giving a choice of what to eat during the day may be what the providers of care consider is good practice, but it may cause considerable irritation to the older person to be asked to choose their meals. Why is this? In the late 1800s or early 1900s, when older people were born and brought up, it was the role of the professionals to know what was best for people, to give them rules by which they should live and to provide for them according to the rules (Fraser, 1995). The professional was also energetic in ensuring the rules were carried out so a carer who

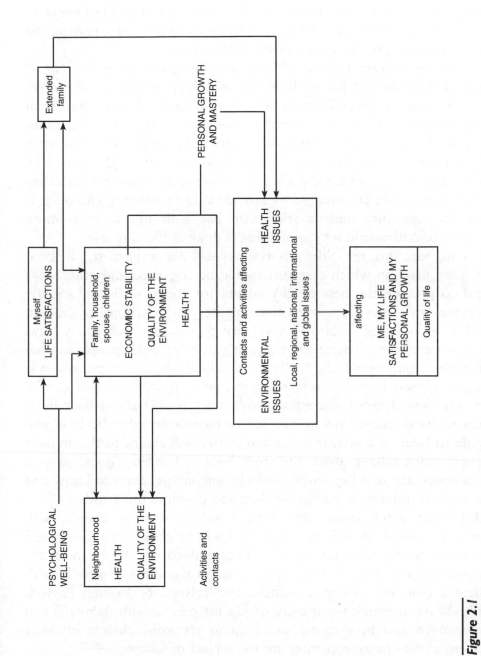

Figure 2.1

Assessing services for older people (adapted from Seed & Lloyd (1997))

asked the patient/client what they wanted was seen to be lacking in knowledge and did not know how to do their job properly! Therefore, it should come as no surprise, given this background, that some older people feel hesitant when asked for their views on a whole variety of aspects affecting their care. In fact, in the eyes of the older person, the carer is undermining their own position by asking.

So, in the current culture of everyone being encouraged to speak about their needs and hopes, how can the older person and the carer come to a compromise? There is no easy solution to this and quality of life is fraught with such dilemmas. However, a good starting point might be for the carer and the older person to begin by talking with each other as friends about what they believe to be the right way to go about things and, from the carer's point of view, the ways in which they are currently being encouraged to provide care by offering choice. It is often the case that once a friendship has built up, there is more readiness to understand why something is done in the way it is.

Having said this, the older person may still not want to speak about what they need, in which case this should be respected and other ways found to provide the best quality of life for them, such as discreetly observing what they appear to like. In the case of choosing food, it could be by noticing (unobtrusively) what they eat and what they leave in a regular pattern. Therefore, providing care for older people implies that carers understand the culture in which the older person was brought up and how this affects their values. A sense of this can be obtained from detailed discussions with older people about their lives, which many of them love to provide to those who take the time and trouble to listen and appear interested in (we will return to this in later chapters when talking about life story books). Current issues, such as the development of a key worker system, encourage carers to know and take a special interest in particular clients to promote this bond.

But what about those who cannot speak, such as people with dementia? Should we still be trying to find out about their needs and hopes? According to quality of life values, indeed we should and there is much ongoing work to find ways to access the views of people with dementia (see, for example, Killick, 1997; Reed & Roskell Payton, 1997). Ways in which the quality of life for people with dementia can be improved and how carers can help to recognise their needs and hopes in a cost-effective manner are the subject of Chapters 4–7.

Second, providing quality of life for older people means that everyone is equal and there should be no sense in which those who need care are in a subordinate position to those who provide the care. This is a further dilemma for care, as many older people are more used to a bureaucracy where those who receive services tend to be at the bottom of the hierarchy. Some older women are also used to being in a subordinate position to both a husband and a father, so therefore will look to men to provide for them and also to speak on their behalf. So, providing quality of care in which those receiving it and those giving it work together on an equal basis may be difficult to achieve.

Third, everyone should have the opportunity to say what their needs and hopes are and have their views respected. Therefore providers of services have been increasingly encouraged to develop a range of ways in which clients can state their views and have them recorded and followed up. These ways include:

- periodic semiformal assessments which are recorded, a copy of which is provided for close relatives;
- residents' meetings at which attendance is not compulsory but minutes of the meetings are kept and resulting action monitored;
- residents' views obtained during inspection visits;
- a complaints procedure which is known to those receiving care as well as to their relatives.

These more formal mechanisms are to support the daily work with clients that carers undertake and in which they gain information about the quality of life of the older person in their care. As well as these systems, some organisations have meetings for relatives and some also organise training for relatives to help them to understand the progress of dementia and so anticipate their relative's likely deteriorating behaviour and condition.

However, these four ways of obtaining clients' views are frequently not conducted on the basis of equality; for example, residents' meetings often discuss the same issues and the staff consistently provide the items for discussion. Given time and if meetings foster a sense of genuinely wanting clients to express their needs and hopes in a relaxed atmosphere, maybe clients will take more of an equal part. But it will be up to staff to promote this equality.

Despite the discussion above about the carer being sensitive to the needs of clients, one of the most enduring features of quality of life is that individuals should have choice. Therefore, in assessment of quality of life, inspectors will undoubtedly be looking to see how choice is given to clients and the range of choice offered in every aspect of service provision.

Due to quality of life values emphasising the promotion of equality between individuals, this section would not be complete without considering the needs and hopes of care workers. As Levering (1994) says:

Quality of life within organisations not only has a major impact on each of us personally but on society as a whole. How we treat each other during our working hours defines what kind of society we have. (p. xxii)

Most carers work for two reasons: financial and altruistic. Satisfaction with rates of pay mainly depends on two factors: the rate that the individual expects for the job; and the comparisons they are able to make with other similar jobs.

While the majority of carers are women, many of whom possess few qualifications and left school early, the rates of pay can be amongst the lowest in the UK. This was pointed out by Dick Clough, General Secretary of the Social Care Association in 1996, when he said:

There's huge financial pressures on independent homes. The payments they are receiving for (state-supported) residents do not allow them to have the same staff backup as in the statutory sector. This has forced the independent sector to pay low rates. (Cervi, 1996, p. 22)

While the independent and voluntary sectors generally pay the lowest rates, council-run homes tend to pay their staff slightly more as well as providing them with local authority terms and conditions. Therefore, local authority homes are often seen by carers as having somewhat better conditions, including pay. In order to keep staff, some private homes have had to offer incentives, for example a pay rise for completed vocational qualifications. The influence of the government's minimum wage on this sector will be bound to have an impact. Also, in nursing homes there are often only two distinct tiers of staff: registered nurses and carers. Therefore, in these homes there is often no potential for promotion, although carers can become workplace assessors for candidates undergoing vocational qualifications.

However, on an altruistic level, many carers express considerable satisfaction with their jobs, particularly if they are in a good organisation and are receiving training, which makes them feel valued as employees, so rates of pay can seem less important. We will return to this in the section on staff training and staff retention on pages 27–29.

Although rates of pay are low, which can affect the quality of life of some carers, particularly single mothers, carers' quality of life is most noticeably threatened when clients are excessively demanding. For example, clients who indicate that the carer should do what they say because they pay their wages are particularly insulting to carers. This is a situation in which managers should intervene to promote the quality of life for the carer. But quality of life for carers will also depend on the numbers of staff. As client:staff ratios are strictly controlled by inspection teams, there is less room for owners to cut staff numbers to compensate for any pay rises put in place by competing organisations or by the government's minimum wage.

However, quality of life for staff of all grades is not usually an area with which inspection teams are concerned, their main concern being the clients (Cervi, 1996). Therefore without government intervention on the minimum wage, these conditions are likely to persist for care assistants.

As we saw from the quotation on page 16, quality of life is also important in providing for the needs and hopes of groups. In the domestic environment, groups are usually already formed as stable units and have often been living together for many years, therefore and have had time to work towards shared needs and hopes. They also frequently have a choice of whom they live with. However, in homes for older people few of the residents have any choice about who else is in the home. Therefore, providing quality of life for groups in nursing and residential homes can be a real challenge as, according to Reed & Roskell Payton (1997), residents build close relationships with some of their peers but they equally loathe others.

Staff are generally very sensitive to which residents get on well together and those that do not. In a large home it is possible to arrange seating during leisure times and at meals so that harmony is promoted. However, in a small home with an emphasis on shared living, particularly if meals are taken together around a single table, there can be considerable friction and a resulting loss of quality of life. This is very difficult for everyone and compromises may be hard to find, although continuing dialogue between carers and residents, if handled sensitively, may help to promote shared understanding.

Where shared rooms are available, choice of a person with whom to share can frequently not be given due to availability. Changes of rooms or sharing a room with someone whose habits are not consistent with one's own can promote acute distress in clients and significantly affect their quality of life.

The final aspect of our definition of quality of life given on page 16 was 'about an individual's personal environment (the setting for their daily living)'. Many of the aspects discussed in the last three paragraphs can also be used in this context. Further factors in the personal environment include the needs and hopes of clients for the state of decoration and comfort of their surroundings. Furniture and fittings that are not only suitable for the person and for which they can feel a sense of ownership, but also which give them a sense of being able to find their way around, make a considerable difference. For new residents and for those in the early stages of dementia, being provided with landmarks and trails to locate essential rooms and spaces can be important to their serenity (we will develop this later in Chapters 5–7).

It is also important for most older people to be able to have a social life outside their immediate surroundings, including being able to sit outside on warm days. So, not only are visitors important but also outings and visits to places of interest as well as holidays can add to stimulation and enjoyment of life for those able to participate.

Quality of life and the principles upon which it is based are as important for older people as they are for everyone else. The values promoted, as defined by Seed & Lloyd (1997), are:

- opportunity;
- choice;
- a positive relationship with the environment;
- non-violent resolution of conflict;
- personal protection;
- respect for everyone's rights;
- openness in dealings with people.

Therefore to live successfully together while being able to develop as an individual is the aim, although this will inevitably involve compromises.

COST EFFECTIVENESS

As we indicated in Chapter 1, cost effectiveness is crucial to staying in business in care, particularly if the majority of clients are funded by the public sector. It is important to put cost effectiveness in its current context, so that we may see how local authorities are currently assessing the cost of services which they purchase.

Following the Labour government's sweeping victory in May 1997, changes to managing and delivering local authority services became evident in the introduction and continued development of 'best value' together with the stated aim of abolishing internal markets, of which compulsory competitive tendering (CCT) was a feature. This was one of the first measures to be introduced by the new government, with announcements being made by the end of May 1997.

Best value is seen to incorporate the principles of CCT, that is, buying services at a competitive price. However, it will no longer be the only management tool; what will also be required are indicators of quality against targets, which were not routinely built into CCT. So, while CCT was seen as effective in driving down costs and in monitoring the performance of contracts, the associated targets on which contracts and performance were based were sometimes not available. There was also said to be no routine continual cycle of improvement. Also, CCT created considerable work in the tendering process and it appears that the Labour government may be abolishing it altogether by April 1999 (Vize, 1997). Best value includes accountability to the public for effective and efficient services with target setting and the measurement of performance against targets. Councils have no requirement to provide services themselves, if more efficient means of providing them are available. 'What matters is what works' (Principle 4 of the Twelve Principles of Best Value). However, competition to provide services will continue and will be set within national standards, which are currently being developed and refined. National standards will allow comparison between authorities on the basis of performance information and will be confirmed by auditors who will report publicly.

Therefore, standards and cost effectiveness of councils will be very public and competitive.

There are a number of implications of this for the care sector. First is the drive by local councils to involve the public more in participating in local affairs. The ways in which councils are developing this approach are varied and many different ways are currently being tried, including citizens' juries – where expert witnesses give their advice to a panel of local people; the development of civic assemblies; and having a number of co-opted members on the main council committees. However, the culture of local government has to change in order for local partici-pation to have a major impact on decision making. Despite this, there is increasing room for local citizens to influence the ways in which decisions about services are made, amongst them services for older people. In this context, local people could also include owners and managers of services for older people.

Second, the development of instruments needed under best value is now moving apace. But are the people who are going to be assessed using these measures, the owners and managers of services for older people, involved in their production and refinement? Also, how valid (that they are measuring what they are supposed to measure) are some of these instruments and who is testing them for validity? This implies a knowledge of rigorous research techniques. Therefore, although openness and equality are two of the main values by which quality of life is defined and services are assessed for older people and these values are increasingly being built into local and national government rhetoric, are they being adopted in drawing up the assessment methods? Or is a predominantly bureaucratic approach still being adopted? Alternatively, as best value demands that councils carry out self-assessment as well as being assessed by external bodies and measured by league tables of performance, this may be such a sensitive area that staff may be working through the implications before developing a more open approach.

However, it is quite difficult to consider cost effectiveness in the care sector, as there are a large number of constraints. These include:

• the income being controlled, as the large majority of clients are referred by the local authority. This appears to be the case even when clients have private means to support their care, as a social work assessment can precede referral which is often then negotiated at local authority rates;

- minimum staffing levels are controlled by being built into contracts and, with the minimum wage, the level of pay for carers will also be maintained;
- overheads, such as routine payments to quality assurance units for inspection, are necessary.

Therefore, how can costs be kept down, apart from routine good house-keeping on expenditure? Management of an organisation would appear to be a key factor in costs, both direct and indirect. Direct costs concern the level of salaries paid to managers, which usually reflects their levels of responsibility, for example the size of the home or the numbers of staff employed/managed. Indirect management costs refer to the level of efficiency by which the organisation operates and by which the effectiveness of management is seen. Barrow & Brown (1997) call this 'leadership' and define it thus:

The essence of visionary leadership lies in two aspects: first articulating the vision or direction of the business, second in mobilising the energies of all the employees towards the vision. (p.94)

Accordingly, they say leadership has three components.

- *The task*: which involves agreeing aims, planning, reviewing and evaluating. In the context of managing the organisation, business planning is recognised as a major part of success in business. Accreditation, such as Investors in People, emphasises the business plan as one of the key features of setting up the structure around which the whole business operates; this also provides a structure for review and evaluation of the organisation. However, many small businesses do not have a business plan, except when required to do so for purposes such as bank loans. Therefore, the performance of the business as a whole is not regularly and systematically reviewed against the objectives. However, although a business planning process may not be in place, systems are in place for clients, as care planning and review are now inbuilt as part of the process of care. Therefore, the ability to plan and review is evident for individuals, but not for the organisation as a whole.

- *The team*: which involves recruiting the right people, communicating with them, encouraging, harmonising and co-ordinating them. It also implies keeping good staff once they have been recruited, as staff recruitment and induction are expensive.
- *The individual*: which involves all the aspects we considered in quality of life, plus training and motivation.

However, these three components cannot be developed in isolation from each other. Linking them in an effective way can help the organisation to be more efficient, to avoid claims of poor-quality care and therefore to be more competitive. Ways of linking the three components have been encouraged in various programmes connected with business development. Those who are either undergoing Investors in People training or have completed the qualification have found that the links between training and the business plan have been useful (Rix, 1994):

> *Internal benefits derived from strengthening links in a loosely connected causal chain. ... Less well organised firms have (also) found benefits in being forced to examine the extent of integration of their training programmes into the overall business plan. Others are taking the opportunity which Investors in People gives them to re-examine the assumptions behind their, perhaps implicit, business plan. (p. 15)*

Therefore, having a workforce which is well trained and co-ordinated, particularly in areas associated with quality of life and its implications for care, and being able to link this to the goals of the business to ensure a smooth and efficient operation should improve the chances of success. It is also likely to improve staff retention and so cut down on recruitment costs. As Levering (1994) says:

> *A great workplace is one where everyone, employees and management, is pulling together. It makes the workers feel better. It makes managers feel better about the roles they play. And it helps society in general. (p. xxii)*

This is clearly quality of life in action for everyone involved. Not only does quality of life make the organisation a very pleasant place to work, the level of harmony also makes it very successful. Also when people are happy at work they carry this feeling of satisfaction home with them at the end of the day. We will develop this further below.

STAFF TRAINING AND STAFF RETENTION

One of the key questions in staff training is whether it makes a difference to the quality of the work the employee undertakes. There is some heartening evidence that it does, although our 'gut reactions' must be that it does. Barron et al. (1997) have shown that particularly in the first three months, on-the-job training makes for a considerable increase in productivity during that period. So, it seems important to have good induction programmes in place that will probably last more than a few hours. It could therefore be very useful to have a form of mentoring for new employees for at least the first three months.

However, on-the-job training cannot be seen in isolation from the rest of the organisation, so we first need to consider what it is like to work in a really good organisation. This might also give us some insight into how to retain staff.

While searching for ways to describe a good organisation from the point of view of employees, I came across a book by Levering (1994) and was immediately enthralled. He describes a good organisation thus:

> From an employee's viewpoint, a great workplace is one in which you trust the people you work for, have pride in what you do, and enjoy the people you are working with. (p. 26) (my emphasis)

He also links this to quality of life. Levering's work was based on inter- views with staff and managers in a large number of organisations in an attempt to define what made a place a great place to work, where employees at all levels said very genuine and positive things about their employers. So the book was not based only on recommendations but also on investigating successful as well as less successful organisations and comparing the two to see what made the difference. He found that employees in 'great places to work' said a number of different things.

• The place was friendly. That the other people are friendly, interesting and will chat informally as an accepted part of everyday life. In such places there is a relaxed atmosphere and everyone appears equal, so nobody has to pretend to be 'busy' or 'important'.

- There were no politics. Due to the atmosphere of mutual respect, people can say what they believe and not fear they will be punished for it; also the management will listen and take action where they can. Employees feel that politicking destroys the sense of working together for a common cause. In such organisations employees are rewarded for being able to work well with others.
- Not being taken advantage of and being treated fairly. This requires a genuine commitment to justice so that employee complaints about being treated unfairly are dealt with and, if necessary, supervisors are overruled and taken to task.
- It's more than just a job. In this kind of place a job has a definite meaning and employees feel it fulfils a definite purpose. This involves having responsibility for what they do and so having a sense of control over their work as well as having a role in defining it and determining the priorities. This fulfils an important social dimension and makes the employee feel proud to be associated with the company. 'Feeling proud of what you do and who you do it with makes people at good workplaces say they have "more than just a job"' (p. 15).
- Work being more like a family. This had a number of very positive aspects to it, such as a caring, nurturing environment where employees feel valued as individuals; workers have a long-term commitment to their jobs and also feel they are 'all in it together', so that everyone plays a distinct and valuable role. This, more than any other, makes employees more productive. However, there is also room within such an organisation for workers who want their privacy and to go home to their families on time. This type of organisation also gives a sense of belonging to the town and community outside the workplace.

This can all sound very idealistic. However, Levering found that the managers and owners in such organisations worked very hard at ensuring equality and a good working atmosphere. Good employers gave a lot of time, energy and thought to the relationships with employees. Trust and having confidence in and relying on their employees were the essential ingredients of the relationship:

Where trust exists, the employer believes the workers want to be productive and participate fully in the enterprise; employees assume the employer has their interests at heart. This trust frees employees to get a deeper sense of fulfilment from their work. (p. 24)

Although this may be seen by sceptics as being rather too good to be true, similar types of conditions have also been found in other studies, such as that of Reynolds & Bruce (1990) looking at staff retention in retailing.

Therefore, merely having staff training in place cannot promote the sense of belonging to a good organisation. The managers need to undergo training themselves, in order to promote harmony in the workforce, a sense of belonging, a satisfying and worthwhile job and a willingness to stay in the job rather than to move to somewhere that appears to offer better conditions. So retention of staff would be likely to improve. It would also be more likely that staff would want to continue to learn about their jobs, as they would take a pride in conti-nuing to improve their performance. When these conditions for employees are considered in the context of the direction of the business, according to the business plan, then everyone pulls together to promote cost effectiveness. It would appear under these conditions that any organisation would be likely to be more competitive. However, in future, all organisations in Scotland will need to train their carers to a recognised level in order to be admitted to a Register, if current proposals become law (The Scottish Office, 1999).

From this review of good management practice in the context of being competitive and successful in business, we turn, in the next chapter, to training. We consider the types of training that are available and how it may be possible to choose between them in the context of caring for older people.

REFERENCES

Barron, J.M., Berger, M.C. and Black, D.A. (1997) *On the Job Training.* W.E. Upjohn Institute for Employment Research, Kalamazoo, Michigan.

Barrow, C. and Brown, R. (1997) *Principles of Small Business*. International Thomson Business Press, London.

Bytheway, W. (1995) *Ageism*. Open University Press, Milton Keynes.

Cervi, R. (1996) Contracting right. *Community Care*, 28 March – 3 April, 22–23.

Fraser, M. (1995) *The History of the Child 1905-1989: How the Child and the Family are Constructed in the Nursing Times*. Unpublished PhD thesis, University of London, Goldsmiths College.

Killick, J. (1997) In their own write. *Community Care*, 15–21 May, 26–27.

Levering, R. (1994) *A Great Place to Work*. Random House, New York.

Reed, J. and Roskell Payton, V. (1997) Privileging the voices of older service users: a methodological challenge. *Social Sciences in Health*, **4**, (4), 230–274.

Reynolds, J. and Bruce, N. (1990) *Recruitment and Retention in Retailing*. Longmans Oxford Institute of Retail Management, Harlow.

Rix, A. (1994) *Investors in People: A Qualitative Study of Employers*. Research Series No. 21. Department of Employment, London.

Schalock, R. (1989). *Quality of Life: Perspectives and Issues*. American Association of Mental Retardation, California.

Seed, P. and Lloyd, G. (1997) *Quality of Life*. Jessica Kingsley Publishers, London.

The Scottish Office (1999) *Striving for Excellence: Modernising Social Work Services in Scotland*. Cm 4288. The Stationery Office, Edinburgh.

Vize, R. (1997) Labour set to scrap CCT in April, 1997. *Local Government Chronicle*, 2 May, 1.

3 TRAINING IN CARE FOR OLDER PEOPLE: THE BIG DEAL

The big deal in the title of this chapter has arisen because organisations caring for older people are being encouraged to train all grades of staff to a recognised level. I do not subscribe to the difference between education and training that is sometimes promoted. Along with Ball (1996), I have come to the view 'that learning for life and learning for work are not easy to separate: (academic) education and (vocational) training have converged' (p.58). Therefore, in the remainder of this book I will refer to education or learning as the means by which we all learn.

As we saw in the last two chapters, no longer is education for care staff an optional extra, it is now being written into contracts with local authorities and is likely to increase in importance in the future. Therefore, organisations need to consider the options for educating their staff, not only in the most cost-effective way possible but also so that education makes a real difference to the care provided. This chapter, then, considers these issues:

1. How can adult education be made relevant to the work so that it is used to continually improve the quality of care?
2. How can education be conducted cost effectively?

This is set against the background of education in care for older people outside the NHS being traditionally something which a few organisations undertook, but these were often the exception. Where education was undertaken it was often only for senior or new staff, so the majority did not receive any form of education or updating on a regular basis and it was considered unnecessary. Where programmes of education were conducted, they were often delivered by the same person who passed on knowledge that they possessed, possibly as a result of a nursing training. However, a senior member of staff would often conduct informal training by working with staff to ensure the care was carried out to their standards but without the senior staff themselves having undergone any updating for a number of years. This form of apprenticeship was often similar to the kind of supervision that student nurses received and was therefore undertaken in a way that emphasised the correct technical skills.

In this context current methods of education have developed. However, in recent years the emphasis on life-long learning and the learning organisation has meant that few people can survive in business or in work without continual learning. I return to this at the end of this chapter and also in the next.

Evidence that learning is now of prime importance has come directly from government, where the consultation paper *The Learning Age* (DfEE, 1998) leaves us no option but to continuously learn:

> *We have no choice but to prepare for this new age in which the key to success will be the continuous education and development of the human mind and imagination.* (p. 9)

Education is no longer an option; we fail to learn and develop at our peril. The price to be paid is to be left behind, which could possibly mean to be unemployable.

HOW CAN EDUCATION MAKE A DIFFERENCE TO THE WORK?

As we noted in the last chapter, most staff work in care for older people because they enjoy it. It can also make a considerable difference if they are receiving education which helps them to recognise that they are doing a good job. But as we all know, education can be delivered in a wide variety of different ways. To be effective, education of adults should take account of their experience; in the case of care workers, this would be their experience of caring for older people, so that it can help them to link their learning with the way they work. In other words, how can education be translated into improving the quality of care? We will look here at adult preferences for education and will then weigh up each of the ways in which it can be delivered, taking into account the cost of each option.

The education of adults has been studied by many people. Some of the leading figures in this field are Jarvis (1983) in the UK, Brockett &

Hiemstra (1991) and Tough (1979) in USA, and Brookfield (1986) in the UK and USA. All these writers agree that life-long learning is here to stay and propose various ways of helping everyone to become life-long learners by assisting them to be self-directed in their learning. Although there are numerous ways of describing self-directed learning, including life-long learning, self-education, self-teaching and independent learning, which have subtle differences, many writers speak of the varying experiences of people who have learnt how to learn and how they came to do it. For example, Brockett & Hiemstra give examples of three people, one who learnt how to study family history, another how to understand and develop alternative sources of power and the third how to take responsibility for her own learning and not to rely on other people giving her information through formal courses of study. The authors describe the excitement and absorption that these people found in learning about things that interest them – not necessarily leading to any formal qualifications, but just for the fun of it, because they found it stimulating. However, Brookfield says that learning to be self-directed may not always be pleasant and may occur as a result of a personal crisis, such as coping with a divorce or experiencing the death of a close relative. In these circumstances, when there is a forced re-examination of ourselves, life can be very unsettling and quite a struggle and uncertainty is frequently felt. Despite this, considerable personal learning and development are almost always part of the process and therefore can equally be called self-directed learning.

What all these writers have in common is that they see adults as having the potential for self-directed learning. In other words, some adults have arrived at a state where they realise what they want to learn and raise questions about what they do not understand. They also know how to get the information they need, to make sense of it when they have it and use it to see if it works before incorporating it into their understanding. This implies that those who are self-directed are able to reflect not only on the initial problem itself but also on the information they have gained so as to assess how useful it is. However, we cannot assume that every adult is like this, far from it, according to Brookfield, who says that learning styles vary considerably from one person to another and depend on a number of factors. However, some of the features that can help the adult to learn appear to include that they want to learn, they have a sufficient level of confidence in their ability to do so and they participate in the learning in a comfortable supportive environment.

The rest of this book will take this approach: that is, considering how senior care staff can become self-directed learners in their care for people with dementia and some of the barriers that will need to be faced if this is to be successful. I want to share with you how I tried to help a group of senior care staff to develop skills of self-directed learning, at their request, and the successes and problems that arose. I hope to suggest how progress can be made towards care workers and managers becoming life-long learners and therefore self-directed in their learning. This approach does not mean that life-long learners will no longer need educators but that learners will be involved in their own education, with educators becoming one of the avenues open to them by providing or suggesting where other resources may be found or helping to direct activities by focusing the problem or discussing alternative methods of seeking solutions.

This approach to adult learning as life-long learning is not new. Many professions are now making it compulsory for their members to update their knowledge and skills; for example, lawyers, doctors, architects and nurses are amongst those groups required to submit evidence of continuing professional development to their professional body in order to maintain their registration to practise in their profession. Self-directed learning leading to life-long learning is now seen as so essential and has become so popular that it is part of everyday language.

In considering how adults may become self-directed learners, Brockett & Hiemstra and Brookfield look at ways in which teachers can help to encourage the learner to learn. They suggest that the teacher and the learner should be much more of a partnership, with the teacher being a resource for the learner so that the learner can increase their control over what and how they learn and not be solely reliant on the teacher to provide the knowledge while they, like a sponge, merely soak it up. This means that the teacher will need to develop ways of helping the learner to identify what they need to know and hope to gain from the knowledge; ways of identifying with the learner where they can find the information they need and how to use it; and then to help the learner to evaluate whether it meets their needs and hopes. So teachers will have to think carefully about how they can help to promote learners' independence before they meet the learners.

As well as the teacher promoting self-directed learning, Brockett & Hiemstra also recognise that there are certain personal characteristics that each person possesses which will need to be taken into account. They say that there is a direct relationship between how good one feels about oneself and how much one goes along with the principles of self-direction or responsibility for one's own learning. Therefore, the barriers within the individual to being a self-directed learner might include negative feelings about oneself such as 'I'm too old' or a lack of confidence or fear of what might result, such as being made to look stupid, all of which hinder the individual's self-development through learning. What these barriers have in common is that they are beliefs that the individual has about their own ability to learn, based on personal perceptions or past experiences or both.

However, when learning takes place in an organisation as part of the work a third factor needs to be taken into account, which is the readiness of the organisation to promote a learning environment. The notion of a learning organisation is relatively new and there is some visionary work ongoing in the area. At the heart of the learning organisation is the idea that groups and individuals are engaged in continuously learning about their work. Marquardt (1997) describes the learning organisation in the following ways:

1. *It is performance based (tied to business objectives).*
2. *Importance is placed on learning processes (learning how to learn).*
3. *The ability to define learning needs is as important as the answers.*
4. *Organisation-wide opportunities exist to develop knowledge, skills and attitudes.*
5. *Learning is part of work, a part of everybody's job description.*
   (p. 180)

Therefore, in this type of organisation everyone is involved in continuously learning about the work and is encouraged and valued for doing so (Mulrooney & Pearn, 1997). Everyone has continuous access to information and resources. Also part of the learning organisation is that change is embraced and the unexpected and even failures are viewed as opportunities to learn. These features are seen as key to the success of the business as, with the current rate of change, it will not be possible for organisations to ignore the pressures of learning.

In the care of older people, part of the push for change and learning will come not only from the pressures of staying in business and being competitive, as we saw from the first two chapters, but also from the need to keep up to date with research into the care for older people. To move towards the learning organisation will be essential.

Therefore, the learner who is likely to be most in tune with directing their own learning will have a combination of the following.

- A belief that they are responsible for their own education and have a specific area of interest which they are highly motivated to develop. They are able to draw on a wide variety of different methods and techniques in order to learn and they have a warm personality with good interpersonal skills and relate well to others. Relating to others is particularly important for those who feel other people are their most important learning resource.
- These personal characteristics combined with a supportive atmosphere provided by a teacher are most likely to promote self-directed learning in those who are at an early stage in developing the skills.
- The organisation in which they work will have a high emphasis on learning during and as part of the work, so that learning and working are one and the same.

These internal and external characteristics can be seen in Figure 3.1.

From Figure 3.1, we can see that in order to arrive at a situation of self-directed learning the organisation must be ready to promote learning in all its activities, the teacher must make a conscious effort to promote self-direction and the learner must also have the characteristics necessary to benefit from the experience, including wanting to develop to become a self-directed learner. Therefore the following guidelines might be offered to any teacher wishing to develop this approach.

1. *Progressively decrease the learner's dependency on the educator.*
2. *Help the learner understand how to use learning resources – especially the experience of others, including the educator, and how to engage others in reciprocal learning relationships.*
3. *Assist the learner to define his/her needs.*
4. *Assist learners to assume increasing responsibility for defining*

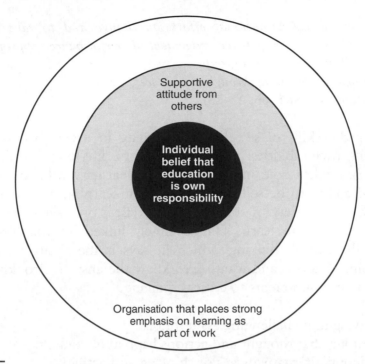

Figure 3.1

Internal and external characteristics which promote self-directed learning

their learning objectives, planning their own learning programme and evaluating their progress.

5. *Organise what is to be learned in relationship to his/her current personal problems, concerns and levels of understanding.*

6. *Foster learner decision making – select learner-relevant experiences which require choosing, expand the learner's range of options, facilitate taking the perspective of others who have alternative ways of understanding.*

7. *Encourage the use of criteria for judging which are different and similar types of learning experiences and can be reflected upon and understood in relation to one's own experience.*

8. *Foster an approach which leads to good quality reflection on learning.*

9. *Facilitate problem posing and problem solving.*

10. *Reinforce the self-concept of the learner as a learner and doer by providing progressive mastery; a supportive climate with feedback*

to encourage provisional efforts to change and to take risks; avoidance of competitive judgement of performance; appropriate use of mutual support groups.

11. *Emphasise learning through experience.*
    (Mezirow, 1981, pp. 22–23).

Promoting the skills of self-directed learning in order to develop the individual's own abilities may well lead to life-long learning. The educator has a key role in promoting the learner's willingness, confidence and ability to be self-directing in their learning by helping them to learn from a variety of sources and to reflect on their experience in order to continue to learn. This is closely linked to what Brookfield (1986) calls 'critical thinking' which he says is the ability to ask why certain things happen and wanting to know the answer. Brookfield says there are four components to critical thinking:

• identifying and challenging assumptions;
• recognising that thought and actions happen in context;
• considering alternative ways of thinking and acting;
• being sceptical – not accepting things because they have always been done that way or because an expert says so.

Critical thinking is closely linked to problem solving, where events cause the self-directed learner to consider paths along which learning may proceed and in which they may involve others; this is not necessarily in a planned manner but can be extremely exciting and absorbing.

One of the reasons why this approach of self-directed learning is important in a care setting is that, as we have said in previous chapters, many staff care for older people because they enjoy the work. Therefore, if they can also learn the skills of learning more about their work by wanting to know more about it and being able to find and use the information they need, then this is likely to increase their enjoyment and motivation and to encourage others to want to be more involved also. What I hoped to create, in the project around which this book is based, was the beginnings of an environment where learning became part of the work, so that the whole organisation evolves to actively support learning, where a culture of learning was normal – the learning environment. In this way learning becomes directly related to the work being undertaken as well as enlivening it. It is expected that this approach will improve the quality of care.

Therefore, it appears that to become self-directed learners, care staff will need to develop the following characteristics:

- be able to reflect on their work with older people and to raise questions about it;
- be able to find information from a variety of sources directly related to the questions they raise;
- to make sense of the information they find;
- try out the information in the situation in which the original questions arose;
- evaluate how this information worked in relation to the questions raised;
- to assess what further information, if any, is needed;
- be encouraged by their organisation to do this on a continuous basis and to encourage others to do the same.

It is expected that everyone will be at different stages of readiness to take on self-directed learning. Becoming a self-directed learner is no easy task but one that I felt was very worthwhile pursuing. The rest of this book will show the strategies used and successes that this approach was able to achieve, along with a critical appraisal of the process and outcomes.

THE DELIVERY OF EDUCATION AND TRAINING – WHAT ARE THE ALTERNATIVES AND WHAT DO THEY COST?

In this section I want to weigh up the possible alternatives in education in care for older people. Bearing in mind the need for us all to become self-directed learners, I will consider how education can not only promote self-direction but also can be cost effective.

The most traditional forms of education are usually through attendance at a course or a series of courses. However, although these are currently widely available from local institutes, colleges and universities, they cannot be guaranteed to: a) give the exact content that each person is looking for in relation to their practice of caring for older people; or b) be such that the information presented can be directly and automatically used in practice; this 'theory–practice gap' is also frequently discussed in relation to nursing (see, for example, O'Connor, 1993).

Undoubtedly the individual is enriched by attending courses but most courses are presented in such a way that generally those attending are not encouraged to seek information for themselves or offered support in trying to do so (Brookfield, 1986). This said, some courses have been specifically designed to promote self-directed learning, but I am not aware of one in the area of care for older people. Therefore, courses will usually give those attending the relevant current knowledge, but as this knowledge becomes out of date further attendance will be needed to be sure that updating is maintained. With the rate of change of knowledge and legislation, this could be a very expensive and time-consuming business, bearing in mind the number of staff that need to undergo basic courses such as moving and handling and first aid.

However, some courses do build in forms of assessment that require students to search for information and to write essays and conduct projects by using the information that they have found. While this teaches students how to find information and to put it together in answer to a specific question, it does not necessarily mean that this information will be used in practice with the care of older people. It also means that the issues that arise as part of work with older people are not necessarily those being answered by the essay or project. The essays and projects may therefore be seen as more of an academic exercise and something to be 'got through' in order to pass the course, rather than a first attempt at learning how to be a self-directed learner in their area of work.

Courses are also traditionally held away from the place of work, although there is evidence that this is changing (Dobson, 1998) and some courses are being held in the workplace. This has considerable benefits; as Dobson has said, it means that the setting in which the work with older people takes place is used in the teaching, so making it more immediately relevant to those attending. However, as information becomes outdated, the course has to be updated and delivered again to those previously attending. Unless there is a form of assessment that requires participants to find information for themselves and make use of it in their work, this form of course delivery will also not lead to self-directed learning. Costs can also be similar to courses in colleges.

Therefore, in course delivery both in the workplace and away from it there is often no requirement for participants to develop skills of self-directed learning. There is also a lack of encouragement in sustained reflection on care for the older person and raising questions about the care, both of which can lead to searching for information. Costs are also recurrent.

A second form of education which has become very popular in the last decade in care of older people is vocational qualifications (VQs and NVQs). These assess what the candidate is currently able to do; in other words, they are outcome measures. They have at least three distinct advantages over conventional courses, as outlined in the above paragraphs:

- candidates have their abilities assessed in their place of work;
- their assessment is conducted during their everyday work with older people;
- candidates have to provide evidence, usually in written form, of the work they have done and relate this to the stated requirements.

This latter requirement means that candidates not only have to do the work satisfactorily, but they also have to reflect on it in order to write about it. The scheme also has the distinct advantage that the people assessing candidates are usually also based in the workplace, so they have to have sufficient knowledge of the requirements in order to assess adequately. This means that everyone is being involved in training.

However, if the candidate does not have the knowledge in order to successfully carry out an activity, then this has to be gained from whatever source is available. The quality of sources can be variable (see Fraser, 1997), as anyone can put on a course. If a traditional course is not available or not at a convenient time then both the candidate and the assessor are challenged to find the knowledge. While the emphasis of VQs is on encouraging the candidate to be self-directed, the way of achieving this is sometimes unclear to both the assessor and the candidate, as is where the necessary knowledge may be found. Therefore, although VQs go a long way towards achieving our objectives of encouraging self-direction in learning as listed on page 39, they have variable success in:

- encouraging candidates and assessors to reflect on their work and to raise questions about it;
- ensuring the information obtained is up to date and directly related to the care being provided;
- ensuring that information obtained is tried out to assess its relevance to the care situation in which the candidate is being assessed.

The cost of VQs themselves is relatively low when taken at face value once a candidate and assessor have had an introduction to what is required, although the costs of assessor induction can be subsidised by the Training Enterprise Councils and Local Enterprise Companies in some parts of the UK. However, costs which are often omitted from calculations are the time of the workplace assessor to assess the candidates as well as the periodic fees for internal and external verification visits. Also, if courses are used to supplement knowledge then costs can mount. It is therefore expensive and also demoralising for homes if candidates leave before completing the qualification, so that not only does the home have to send others on induction courses to replace those that have left but they also do not receive any benefit from the training in which they invested.

A third alternative to promoting an organisation in which carers and managers are self-directed incorporates the principles of setting aims, taking action and evaluating the effects of the action in order to assess the direction and goals that form the next stage. This approach is known as action research (AR). The best definition of action research I have found is:

> ... *the study of a social situation with a view to improving the quality of action within it*. (Elliott, 1991, p.69)

As the above quotation indicates, the approach is based on considering which actions need to undergo change and the focus then becomes the changes that are necessary. AR has been widely used in education and it is currently popular in health and social care. It can build on VQs, as indicated above, and can be used in conjunction with them but encourages more of a self-directed approach in which the teacher and those seeking knowledge form a partnership. The principles of this approach in health and social care are developed in Hart & Bond (1995). This approach is briefly described here and its advantages over the other two methods described above are outlined. The next chapter will show why this approach was important in working with a group of eight nursing and residential homes.

In this approach, what is to be learnt is agreed between the learner and the teacher through negotiation and discussion and forms the aims of learning. The teacher does not necessarily have the knowledge or the answers but can help by suggesting where they may be found. As part of the aims, the way in which the information can be obtained and who is going to obtain it are also negotiated. Once the information is found it is discussed and both parties assess how useful it is in relation to the original aims. By trying out the information in the situation that originally provided the aims, both the learner and the teacher are able to see how well it works and what else needs to be understood. This process is shown in Figure 3.2.

Therefore, this approach is geared towards making changes by taking

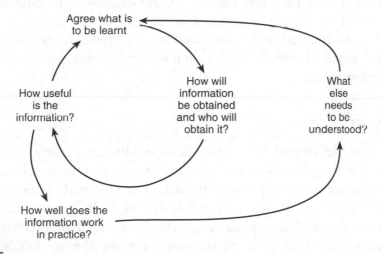

Figure 3.2

The process of teaching/facilitating self-directed learning

action to achieve one or more aims, evaluating the effects of the action and setting new goals. Using this approach, it is possible to critically assess the process by reflecting on what has been achieved and the ways in which these achievements have been reached and also, probably more importantly, to consider a number of influences that made an impact on these achievements, including the backgrounds of the people involved and the culture in which the care for older people is delivered, and how these help to promote a learning environment.

The approach I adopted was to help key senior care staff to become self-directed so that once the project was completed and I withdrew, they could continue to be self-directed. This would help with the development of their staff who were undergoing VQs as well as their own continued development. In considering this approach as the most cost effective, I took into account that each organisation had one or more assessors for VQs already in place. These assessors, although having a good level of knowledge themselves, could not be expected to be up to date in every area they were to assess. It was therefore important for them to continually improve their knowledge so that they could give the best judgements on their candidates' performance. In becoming self-directed learners, it was expected that these key staff would be developing themselves and their organisation while also caring for the residents/clients. The costs of learning would be contained within the staff budget of the organisation, although there would need to be an allowance made for occasions when material needed to be located and assimilated from outside. It therefore seemed that this approach would have a number of benefits, one of which was cost containment.

SUMMARY

I have now developed the approach of self-directed learning which can lead to life-long learning and the learning organisation, in relation to the development of senior staff in care of people with dementia. I have also looked at various ways in which this might be approached and the benefits and problems of each approach. This chapter concluded by introducing the idea of a partnership between the teacher and those wanting to pursue a particular topic and how this might be taken forward. The next chapter gives the principles of this approach in more detail and leads into the following chapters which describe the project and how it was set up, along with its outcomes, in detail.

REFERENCES

Ball, C. (1996) Learning organisations and lifelong learners – the shape of things to come in the learning society. Town and Gown lecture, University of Strathclyde.

Brockett, R.G. and Hiemstra, R. (1991) *Self-Direction in Adult Learning.*: Routledge, London.

Brookfield, S.D. (1986) *Understanding and Facilitating Adult Learning.* Open University Press, Buckingham.

Department for Education and Employment (1998) *The Learning Age.* Cm 3790. The Stationery Office, London.

Dobson, K. (1998) Delivering NVQs on site to care assistants. *E.A.G.L.E. Supplement* **1**, 1.

Elliot, J. (1991) *Action Research for Educational Change.* Open University Press, Milton Keynes.

Fraser, M. (1997) Editorial. *Social Sciences in Health*, **3**, 1.

Hart, E. and Bond, M. (1995) *Action Research for Health and Social Care: A Guide to Practice.* Open University Press, Buckingham.

Jarvis, P. (1983) *Adult and Continuing Education: Theory and Practice.* Croom Helm, London.

Marquardt, M. (1997) Building the learning organisation – examples of good practice. *Lifelong Learning in Europe*, **3**,179–186.

Mezirow, J. (1981) A critical theory of adult learning and education. *Adult Education*, **32**(1), 3–24.

Mulrooney, C. and Pearn, M. (1997) The chicken and the egg: lifelong learning and the learning organisation. *Lifelong Learning in Europe*, p. **2**, 76–81.

O'Connor, H. (1993) Bridging the gap? *Nursing Times,* **89**(32), 30–31.

Tough, A.M. (1979) *The Adult's Learning Projects: A Fresh Approach to Theory and Practice in Adult Learning.* Ontario Institute for Studies in Education, Toronto.

4 COMBINING AIMS, ACTION AND EVALUATION IN PRODUCING CHANGE

This chapter continues where Chapter 3 finished. I want to analyse in more detail what action research (AR) can do and why it is important in a situation such as helping senior care staff to understand more about care for their clients with dementia. To start, it is crucial to understand the values incorporated in AR and how these are consistent with modern ideas of care for older people in community settings. In the second part of the chapter I will develop some of the issues in setting up an action research project so that participation in change may be achieved.

UNDERSTANDING THE VALUES UNDERPINNING THE APPROACH

Action research has its base in education and has been developed since the 1940s. Its principles are concerned with six main issues, as developed by Winter (1987).

- The topics are concerned with professional knowledge but reflecting on it, and the judgements made, will raise questions about the professional knowledge.
- The practical experience of those involved is used as the basis for transforming their actions by recognising the possibilities for alternative courses of action.
- By reflecting on their actions, the personal interpretations of those involved will be made clear as will the consequences of these interpretations.
- Those involved in the process will undergo change themselves, due to their reflection on their practice and the context in which it takes place, as they make changes in their practice.
- There may well be contradictions between those involved and

negotiation may not mean that a consensus among all parties is reached.

- There are two levels of question – the question of practice by theory and the question of theory by practice. Therefore by comparing theory and practice and changing actions accordingly, which will lead to further questions, everyone will have their practice changed.

Becoming more critical of one's own actions and so becoming more self-aware increases the self-esteem of those who participate in learning through experience. It is therefore a process where participation in raising awareness and consciousness of issues have been the main themes. Hart & Bond (1995), who work in a health and social care context, say:

> ... *much contemporary action research in social care and education (is) 'awareness-raising' and 'consciousness-raising' (and) ha(s) displaced 're-education'.* (p. 49)

Due to the nature of participation, those involved have to be active in the process in order to learn and for change to occur; therefore merely sitting in a classroom listening to a teacher is seen as insufficient to produce change in actions and in values. It is also implicit that empowering of participants takes place; in other words, participants learn how to take more responsibility for themselves and for their learning. As self-directed learning and the learning organisation are now such strong features of our society, as we saw from the last chapter, an approach where participants are encouraged to take responsibility for their own learning is entirely appropriate.

However, in social life in general we must acknowledge political forces, so in any attempt to promote learning and the associated changes in practice there will be positive forces and negative forces. In care establishments, the current emphasis on learning and obtaining qualifications being promoted by inspection teams is one of the positive forces, while another is the enjoyment of the work expressed by most of those caring for older people. Two of the negative forces must be the bureaucracy and the ethos of 'getting through the work', where education is less important, that some organisations demonstrate. It is no great surprise that these two opposing dimensions came through loud and clear in the project discussed in the next two chapters. The organisations involved in the project were not unusual; their approach and level of involvement possibly cover the entire range of responses to promoting self-directed learning in most care settings. These responses were clearly evident in the tussles that staff appeared to experience in some of the institutions that were involved.

Action research is also known to create tensions as changes of actions are the aims. As Greenwood (1994) has pointed out, there are two levels at which change will take place, which are like peeling an onion. The top layer is where changes in actions take place because participants learn that a different way might bring better results. However, this can destabilise the status quo (the second layer of the onion) and bring about a backlash from other people and from the organisation as a whole, therefore rendering the initial action and the person performing it very vulnerable. Instead of increasing their self-esteem, this reaction can lessen it. A simple example of this would be the use of lotions and potions in the treatment of pressure sores, where egg white and oxygen (yes, this practice does still go on!) is replaced by turning to relieve pressure. Unless those in a senior position agree with such a change and endorse its use, their wrath at the person suggesting it could turn other members of staff against the person making or suggesting the change. This is not only because a more junior member of staff has attempted to overturn established practice but also because the practice has been challenged and, with it, the values of those carrying out the practice who are now seen to be out of date. Therefore, Greenwood warns against novices rushing in with missionary zeal to conduct AR without considering the possible consequences.

There are two other political forces that will also be evident in using a participative approach to learning: what Hart & Bond refer to as either the 'professionalizing' strategy or the 'empowering' strategy. By the professionalizing strategy, they mean that the groups that aspire to professional status, such as nursing, teaching and social work, wish to enhance their status by increasing their levels of education in order to have control over their work, including the development of research-based practice (this is seen in the six points developed by Winter on pages 47, 48). In a professionalizing strategy, how work is conducted will be defined by the professional group in negotiation with the users.

Furthermore, the kinds of actions taken at work will be the way in which problems are defined by reflecting on practice and the experience of work; progress and improvement will also be defined by the practitioners on behalf of the users. Therefore the control over work, including the type of knowledge needed to carry it out, and how the work is to be conducted and evaluated belong to the professional group itself; an example of this might be nurses deciding what is the best treatment for clients based on evidence from research, rather than relying on doctors to tell them what to do.

In the 'empowering' strategy, the balance of power shifts from the researcher to the participants, who share the control of the research process by participating in it; they are then empowered to act on their own behalf. It is centred on creating self-confidence, self-expression and an interest in learning. Becoming empowered enables the individual to say with confidence what they feel, like, think and want (Inglis, 1997). As the Participatory Research Network (1982) defined:

> *Participatory research is a tool which oppressed people can use to begin to take control of the economic and political forces which affect their lives ... Control ensures that the new knowledge created arises from their own experience, relates to their perceived needs and is used for their own benefit.* (Cited in Joyappa & Martin, 1996, p. 3)

In this approach the understanding of situations is the subject of discussion between all involved and the outcomes and definitions of improvement are agreed; an example of this might be negotiation with care staff about how, where and when they wish to be assessed for VQs and what will be sufficient for them to be assessed as competent. Therefore an empowering approach is closely linked to ways of changing events, where the researcher takes the role of change agent. It is often open ended and the process is more important than the outcome. It is an approach which has been used with community groups to explicitly address the imbalance of power of vulnerable groups, such as those in poverty. However, as might be assumed from the nature of negotiation, there can often be conflict which has to be worked through in order for a way forward to be found, but this does not mean that everyone necessarily agrees. I found the empowering strategy highly relevant in working with senior care workers; however, I found the terminology used in academic texts, which described participants as being 'oppressed', offensive. In an approach which places such strong emphasis on shared and negotiated understandings, I was surprised that this term was so frequently used in case studies of projects. As I hope some of those who formed part of this project will read this work, I have specifically refrained from using this term, as I did not ever hear any of the participants or the clients with whom they work describe themselves in this way, despite the fact that they are low paid and often lack qualifications.

As well as the professionalising strategy being consistent with increased levels of education for all staff in care for older people, the empowering strategy is vital in helping senior carers, and also the older people for whom they care, to have more of a say in their work and in their lives. Apart from obtaining a qualification taken over a lengthy period of time, I have not found that attending courses has this effect. I mentioned in Chapter 1 that carers were often women with low levels of education, so for them empowerment may be very appropriate. Therefore both of these strategies (professionalizing and empowerment) were used in combination in the project which forms the next two chapters. For all these reasons, action research was seen as an ideal method by which to develop the project of teaching senior carers about care for people with dementia.

AR also allowed for a rigorous analysis of the process and outcomes of the project, so that we may all learn from what was achieved – and what was not achieved!

SETTING UP A PARTICIPATORY PROJECT TO ACHIEVE CHANGE

This section will deal with issues arising in the early days of setting up an action research project in order to promote change. As will be realised from the first part of this chapter, it is not possible to plan an AR project from beginning to end before the start, as reflection on action followed by changes and further reflection (evaluation) on how these changes have worked are the nature of such a project. The next two chapters describe how I used these strategies in the project and show how it developed with senior care staff in helping them to participate in and reflect on how to care for their residents with dementia.

A number of issues need to be considered in participation to promote change. The first of these is the role of the researcher themselves. Sometimes someone outside the organisation is asked in to lead the work but there can be resistance to this and sometimes even outright refusal to let them into the organisation, despite numerous efforts and a great deal of patience, as Kendall & Sturt (1996) found. Therefore negotiating access to conduct the work can be considerably time consuming and without any certainty of success. However, there are many accounts of successful intervention in health by someone from outside the organisation, particularly where they are invited in. For example, in three projects conducted by Hart & Bond (1995, pp. 81–102, 103–122, 147–162), they were outside researchers being asked to develop and participate in the projects. Despite being asked in to develop a project, the outsider always risks being asked to stop the project if they produce unacceptable results, as Hart found. Therefore, once in the organisation, continual negotiation at a number of different levels may need to occur in order for progress to be made. There will also sometimes be pressure to produce the results that the organisation wants; therefore, for the researcher to remain unbiased can also take courage, skill in negotiation and often patience, while bearing in mind that if participants choose poor options, despite knowing the results of their choice, then their rights to choose must be respected. Street (1998) found such a situation when negotiating shift patterns with nurses, where they made choices that were likely to lead to poor health, despite knowing the implications of their choice. This type of situation clearly shows the sort of conflicts that might arise in an empowering approach.

However, it is also possible to promote change through participation by working inside the organisation, as Bond has shown in two further case studies (Bond, 1982, 1990; Hart & Bond, 1995). Working from inside an organisation has the advantage of knowing the situation and the people involved well from the outset; however, being an insider does have disadvantages. Whereas someone from inside an organisation does not have the problems of access, it is often difficult, as an insider, to conduct such work due to the need to divorce oneself from being a work colleague and to take on a more objective role in relation to the project. The switch from project leader to manager or worker can be stressful and at times it is all too easy to give up. Those who have worked inside an organisation while conducting such a project have often found it necessary to discuss issues and progress with someone outside, in order to maintain their objectivity (see Lofland & Lofland, 1995). This can also help to alleviate the sense of isolation some project leaders feel.

Apart from the role played by the person who wishes to promote change, deciding on who and how many are going to be involved in the change needs to be carefully considered. It is often not possible, nor is there sufficient time to involve everyone in the organisation directly so a choice has to be made about who to include directly in the project. While those at the top of an organisation need to be in agreement that this type of change is needed, they may not necessarily be those who are most involved with the process. However, it is vital to achieve their commitment to the aims in order for changes to be able to occur and to be promoted throughout the organisation. It is also unlikely that those at the bottom of a hierarchy will be able to make significant changes on their own, without support from more senior people with sufficient knowledge of what they are trying to achieve. Therefore, it may be better to identify key people who are in a position to make a significant impact on those at the top of the organisation, while also being able to promote change by discussion and persuasion with those with whom they work.

Setting up the project so that all are in agreement with the broad aims and the negotiated roles they will play will be an important step, although flexibility is essential if successful negotiation and participation are to continue as the project unfolds. Also, the timescale over which the project will run must be agreed at the outset, particularly if there are financial limits. However, AR projects cannot be planned very far ahead because, as I have said above, as projects unfold original questions are often reformulated, the focus shifts and new questions emerge (Biott, 1996).

While these three stages (the role of the researcher; who is involved and setting up the project) may sound straightforward, they frequently take many months and involve numerous negotiations, depending on the number and size of the organisations involved. It may also be necessary, in organisations that have ethics committees, to obtain ethics committee agreement to the project being undertaken. Therefore, time and patience are of the essence in achieving a satisfactory start. However, in successful projects using this approach, not only will knowledge be gained but also practice will change due to the participatory nature of the learning and the knowledge being identified in order to provide answers to real questions and problems. More important than this is the method of learning which will change from one where knowledge is seen to exist outside the individual and is accessed by attending courses in order to learn that knowledge, to one where the individual has responsibility for questioning their own practice, weighing up the alternative answers and then trying them out to evaluate how the change worked in practice.

A participatory approach, such as described above, will enable knowledge gained to be used, retained and developed in the organisation for everyone's benefit. AR is therefore closely linked to learning how to learn by reflection and action and can involve the whole organisation in learning. These are considerable advantages over attendance at conventional courses.

SUMMARY

In this chapter we have developed the principles behind action research (AR) and how it can be used to promote reflection on actions which lead to changes in practice and evaluation of the effectiveness of these changes. This will lead to an increasingly professional approach to work, where those involved take responsibility for their own development and also increase their self-esteem in the process. As I have mentioned elsewhere (Fraser, 1996), this is what Schon (1983, 1987) has called reflection in action and is the process professionals can achieve in their practice.

In this chapter I have also evaluated some of the work that needs to be achieved before a project can begin, indicating some of the problems that may arise. The next two chapters will show how the principles developed so far have been used in a project with senior care staff in caring for their clients with dementia.

REFERENCES

Biott, C. (1996) Latency in action research: challenging perspectives on occupational and researcher identities. *Educational Action Research*, 4, 2, 169–183.
Bond, M. (1982) *Women's Work in a Woman's World: The Home Help Service*

Re-examined. University of Bristol School for Advanced Urban Studies, Bristol.

Bond, M. (1990) *Medication Matters: Improving Medication Practices in Residential Homes for Older People.* University of Warwick and SCA, Coventry.

Fraser, M. (1996) *Conceptual Nursing in Practice.* 2nd edn. Chapman and Hall, London.

Greenwood, J. (1994) Action research: a few details, a caution and something new. *Journal of Advanced Nursing,* **20,** 13–18.

Hart, E. and Bond, M. (1995) *Action Research for Health and Social Care: A Guide to Practice.* Open University Press, Buckingham.

Inglis, T. (1997) Empowerment and emancipation. *Adult Education Quarterly,* **48,** 1, 3–17.

Joyappa, V. and Martin, D.J. (1996) Exploring alternative research epistemologies for adult education: participatory research, feminist research and feminist participatory research. *Adult Education Quarterly,* **47,** 1, 1–14.

Kendall, S. and Sturt, J. (1996) Negotiating access into primary health care using action research: insights from critical theory. *Social Sciences in Health,* **2,** 2, 107–120.

Lofland, J. and Lofland, L. (1995) *Analysing Social Settings: A Guide to Qualitative Observation and Analysis.* Wadsworth, Belmont, California.

Schon, D. (1983) *The Reflective Practitioner.* Temple Smith, London.

Schon, D. (1987) *Educating the Reflective Practitioner.* Jossey-Bass, San Francisco.

Street, A. (1998) From soulmates to stakeholders: issues in creating quality postmodern participatory research relationships. *Social Sciences in Health,* **4,** 2.

Winter, R. (1987) *Action Research and the Nature of Social Inquiry: Professional Innovation and Educational Work.* Avebury, Aldershot.

5 SETTING UP THE LEARNING ENVIRONMENT FOR CARE OF OLDER PEOPLE WITH DEMENTIA

INTRODUCTION

In this chapter I will discuss the way in which the project was set up to help senior care staff to become self-directed learners in caring for their clients with dementia. This discussion will include the reasons for the project, the contents of the programme according to the negotiated needs and the role I played, as an outsider, in the project. I will also discuss the people involved, although they will be anonymised, in order to give a flavour of their particular needs and also to show that they had a broad array of different requirements and came from a wide variety of organisations. These organisations probably cover most of the range of services currently offered to older people. The involvement of different organisations occurred because of existing contacts that I had, rather than being specifically planned to incorporate such a mix.

After every contact and following the initial two days of teaching I made copious field notes, in line with Lofland & Lofland (1995) and Burgess (1991). This was for two reasons: in order to remember the needs of the individuals involved for follow-up in each of the organisations, and with a view to later analysis in more detail.

THE INITIAL CONTACT

A manager whom I knew well, of a small church home, telephoned me to say that he was having real difficulty with one of his residents who was showing signs of dementia. This was upsetting the rest of the residents, particularly at mealtimes (all residents ate their meals together around a single table). Knowing how all the other residents were fit and active, I assumed that the disruption was being vocally indicated to the manager. I knew this home and the manager well as I had been asked to conduct some previous teaching in the home. The manager asked me how I could help, indicating that he wanted an intensive programme in care of people with dementia. Having given this some thought, I considered that such a programme might be of interest to other homes as well. However, I was not happy to merely give classroom-based teaching, as I was concerned that this may not lead to much change in behaviour. As a nurse, a qualified nurse teacher and an academic, my position had always been to make education relevant to practice. Therefore my background has a considerable bearing on the approach I preferred to take and on which I negotiated with the other organisations I contacted.

With these initial thoughts I went to see the manager who had contacted me to discuss ideas of having some initial teaching in the principles of dementia, followed by a set number of hours in which I would work with staff in individual homes to look for solutions to some of the problems they were experiencing. He again specified he wanted an intensive course and agreed with these initial thoughts, as well as the aim of getting a few other homes to participate. We agreed that the course should be for senior staff who had responsibility for education of carers, as this was the level that would be most influential in promoting changes in care.

Coincidentally one of the inspectors from the local quality assurance unit indicated to me that homes needed to know more about dementia care mapping, as this was now becoming very popular with inspection teams. Further discussion with the home who made the initial inquiry confirmed that this was, indeed, an element we should include in the programme.

I contacted a further 13 organisations who cared for older people to ask if they would be interested in considering such a programme. Six of the organisations agreed to participate and a further organisation said they could not participate at the moment, but would like to be involved in a future programme. By this time, due to the numbers involved, I had to specify that we could only take three people per organisation. Further contacts at the local college, with whom I had done some work, provided one further organisation who wished to participate (organisation E below). In costing the programme we were able to make use of funds from the local enterprise company.

THE ORGANISATIONS INVOLVED

The participants were eight organisations spread over a 30-mile radius.

- Organisation A was a long-term private residential home for care of older people. It had recently opened a new wing. Its care staff were undergoing VQs at level II and III. Its owner, who was also heavily involved in running the home, participated with two of her senior care staff.

- Organisation B was a voluntary organisation providing domiciliary support for all age groups. They had a part-time trainer who was assessing VQs to level II. Their trainer participated.

- Organisation C was a long-term private residential home for older people, which had just opened a new, purpose-built wing for people with dementia. They were involved in training their care staff to VQ level II. Two of their senior care staff involved in the new dementia wing participated.

- Organisation D was a long-term care residential home. They were part of a consortium to undertake VQs, but progress had been slow. Three of their senior care staff participated.

- Organisation E was a purpose-built long-term church home for people with dementia. They had a full-time trainer as part of their staff and had an extensive training programme for staff and also included relatives. The full-time trainer and two senior care staff participated. I did not know this home and its participants before the programme started.

- Organisation F was a private residential home for care of older people. They said they did not have any residents currently with dementia but would like to learn about it. They were part of a consortium to undertake VQs but progress had been slow. Two of their senior care staff participated.

- Organisation G was a private nursing home for care of older people with a day centre attached. They were involved in VQ training at levels II and III and had made good progress. Their matron, deputy matron and one of the senior care staff participated.

- Organisation H was a small church residential home. They were assessing VQs at levels II and III. Their two joint managers participated.

The total number of participants was 19. As can be seen from the above list, their levels of experience in care of people with dementia, as well as their experience in training their staff was very varied. I had good knowledge of all the organisations and most of the staff that attended, apart from organisation E and its participants.

THE PROGRAMME

As it became clear who was going to be involved, I was able to further refine the type of programme and to negotiate this with each organisation individually by telephone to reach an agreement. It was not possible to arrange a joint meeting to discuss this with all organisations together, but individual negotiation did not create a problem. From the initial telephone call to final agreement of the aims, date and initial content of the programme took a number of weeks.

We agreed that the programme would have two intensive days of teaching which would include aspects of dementia care mapping (DCM) according to a literature search of the area. In undertaking DCM I used a combination of literature produced by Kitwood (1990a, b, 1991–2, 1992) and Kitwood & Bredin (1992) as well as more philosophical work by Graham (1992).

We were able to use a room in one of the local colleges for these two days. This would be followed by 8 hours in each organisation when I would work with the participants. These 8 hours would be to look at the problems they were experiencing with their individual clients with dementia and how we all might learn to understand their needs better.

THE EXPRESSED NEEDS OF THE PARTICIPANTS

At the beginning of the two days of intensive teaching I gave each participant a sheet to complete (which was anonymous, although five participants included their name) on which I asked them to indicate their needs for education in care for people with dementia (a copy of this precourse information sheet is included as Appendix 2). This was intended for my use only as a guide to the expressed education needs of participants. I indicated this to the participants before I gave the sheets out for completion.

Analysing the precourse responses according to Watson (1997) using

However, three of the participants felt training, or the lack of it, was an issue: one of these gave her 2 years of training in 2 different organisations before stating her experience, evidently feeling she had been properly prepared for working with people with dementia. The other two participants referred to psychiatric training, as a nurse, being important:

Worked in psychiatry in NHS for 11 years.

I have worked in the 'care of the elderly' environment for several years without the experience of psychiatric training.

The second quotation suggests that the participant feels that psychiatric training would have been an advantage in caring for her clients, particularly as this is the first statement she made in response to the question 'What is your experience of people with dementia?' Also, I knew of the view within this organisation that a member of staff with psychiatric training would have been an advantage, due to the number of clients they had with dementia. However, both the above participants indicated that they had come into contact with people with dementia, suggesting that they had not really learnt anything from this experience but that it had been part of the work. This view of not having sufficient knowledge despite having worked with clients with dementia for a number of years is reflected by a participant working in organisation D, who said that after 20 years she had 'some experience of their needs', indicating that it is possible even after this length of time still not to fully understand their needs or how to care for them.

Two participants were sufficiently familiar with the professional understanding of dementia to refer to people with dementia as 'p.w.d'. So, despite one of them saying she 'felt inadequate in my knowledge of the disease and how to deal with it appropriately' she evidently had come into contact with professional terminology in the field of dementia. It is also noteworthy that this person referred to dementia as a 'disease', taking a medical approach to the condition. A further participant from the same organisation (G – a nursing home) also used a medical expression by writing that 'dementia had presented itself'.

Six of the participants showed knowledge of the different stages of dementia in such phrases as 'severe dementia', 'later stages of dementia', 'many different stages' and 'some with mild some with moderate and the four questions on the precourse information sheet provided the background to the participants' felt needs and where they placed themselves according to the social order of which they were a part. Watson's analysis is entirely appropriate as he saw written materials influencing the actions of the reader (me) and the writer (the participants); he also saw the reader of the materials combining their own understanding with actions to fully interpret the writing. Responses to the precourse information sheet are grouped according to their similarity as interpreted by me and discussed with participants on my visits to their organisations. There was 100% agreement with my interpretations.

What is your experience of people with dementia?

Responses to the first question 'What is your experience of people with dementia?' varied considerably. The least experience was virtually nothing: 'Very little' and 'Nothing much' were all that was written by both participants from organisation F. These comments were similar to those made by them in negotiating the programme. However, despite their lack of experience, they clearly recognised the importance of an understanding of dementia or they would not have attended, as there was no suggestion that they had been 'sent' by their organisation.

From the other 17 responses, 11 stated the number of years they had worked with people with dementia; the least experienced was 18 months while the most experienced was 20 years. Four of these participants gained experience previously by working in NHS hospitals. Two participants mentioned working with their current clients only and did not include a history of caring for people with dementia. Apart from clients with dementia, four participants had cared for relatives with dementia and so had very personal experience. However, three of these participants assessed their experience with relatives as less important than experience in a care setting where they were paid employees.

Eight of the participants gained their experience from working with people with dementia; for example:

I have worked with dementia sufferers for over eight years and gained experience in many areas of how to cope with different situations.

This participant from organisation E feels that her main experience has been gained from working with clients, rather than from courses.

occasionally severe dementia'. It was also evident that one participant was familiar with different 'types of dementia'; she worked in organisation E (a specialist home for care of people with dementia). She also described care as 'treating them all as individuals', so displaying a recognition of individual differences in approaches to care.

Two of the participants indicated that they felt their role was to care not only for the people with dementia but also for their relatives. One of these worked in a domiciliary environment (organisation B) while the other worked in a specialist dementia unit attached to a private residential home (organisation C). She saw her role as:

helping the families come to terms with the increasing dependence of their relatives or spouses and providing care and support to both parties.

This was despite her claims of experience of only three years in care for people with dementia.

One further response from a participant from organisation C was that in caring for older people over a number of years she had 'of course' come into contact with people with dementia. This indicates that she knew that dementia was so common that if you worked with older people for any length of time, you were bound to come across it. Another participant said that previous people with dementia had been 'very elderly' and 'frail' implying that they were not active or uncontrollable. However, one of her clients who clearly made an impression on her was:

a fit and active lady who was in the later stages of dementia, I was exhausted after one shift and so were our other residents.

Therefore this lady had severely disrupted the serenity of the organisation of 'very elderly' and 'frail' residents and had left staff unable to understand or control her.

Two further responses were about the necessity of special accommodation for people with dementia:

This lady is now in a closed unit.

This statement was made by the same person about two different clients and was clearly a reflection of people with dementia needing secure accommodation well away from everyone else. It has overtones of incarceration. The reason that this was felt to be necessary was the great stress that dementia put on the staff because both these clients needed 'one-to-one' care and 'need(ed) ... care day and night' which she felt unable to give with the existing staff on duty in a small home (organisation H).

What did you feel like looking after these people with dementia?

The second question on the precourse questionnaire was 'What did you feel like looking after these people with dementia?' Apart from one participant, who had indicated in the first question that she had 'nothing much' in terms of experience, the other 18 participants varied widely in their comments. Four participants described feeling 'frustrated' that they could not do more or did not know how to deal with situations; one of these participants also said she did not know how to occupy the clients' time.

Further feelings that affected the participants included sadness, inadequacy, hopelessness and helplessness, as expressed by one participant:

> *There are many occasions when one feels so helpless when a person is really agitated and has to be on the move all the time.*

This was from someone working in a specialist unit for care of people with dementia who had seven years experience in this kind of work. Similar feelings were expressed by six of the participants and included being saddened at the destruction of the person and difficulty in understanding what the person needed. The first of these comments (about destruction of the person) showed knowledge of the processes of dementia. Another of the participants went further and said she felt 'often bruised both physically and mentally', indicating a deep feeling of uncertainty and personal harm. This participant was from organisation D who said she had worked with people with dementia for 20 years.

However, three of the participants said their negative feelings only arose initially and that since then they had learnt through courses and experience and now felt more confident. All three had different lengths of experience of people with dementia, from 7 to 13 years. Further negative feelings that affected two of the participants were that the work was intense and tiring; one of the participants said that combined with trying to care for other residents, caring for the person with dementia 'became a 24-hour day'. Therefore her role had changed from one that was contained in a normal shift pattern, with her other residents, to one where she was performing her role every hour of the day and night. In this home (organisation H) there was a sleep-over arrangement for care staff, as most of their residents slept all night every night, so separate night duty staff were not used. This participant was clearly aware that sedating a client with dementia may well produce a satisfactory outcome for staff, but not necessarily for the person with dementia, as she said it would:

> ... *help the quality of life for that client, without her being over-drugged.*

While this shows regard for the client's quality of life, it also shows that drugs form a regular and well-known means of sedating clients as a way of providing care, although a balance needs to be struck. This participant also said that she 'needed to care, and help', indicating more of a sense of duty and possibly it being a woman's role, rather than any sense of pleasure in the experience. Despite these negative comments, only two participants mentioned levels of stress, one saying 'High levels of stress are felt by all staff caring for dementia residents'. However, this was in a new unit (organisation C) which had opened within the last few weeks, where all the residents were new and feeling unsettled and the staff were becoming accustomed to new roles and surroundings.

One further comment was that one participant felt 'very unprepared and untrained, despite having an HNC care qualification'. This shows disenchantment with a course that did not give 'the answer' to caring for these kinds of clients; it gives the impression of wanting a 'quick fix' rather than a sustained period of learning through experience combined with courses and shows a certain desperation about knowing what to do for these clients. Two participants also mentioned the relatives and family 'coming to terms with' the person with dementia; one of these indicated that the changes in the person as a result of dementia were happening in front of their (the relatives') eyes.

There were equal numbers of positive comments about caring for people with dementia, although some were less enthusiastic than others.

One less enthusiastic comment was that, given time and regular contact with the same people with dementia, it is possible to recognise their behaviour patterns, although not to understand them. This was reflected by another participant who indicated that it was easier to care for people with dementia if you had cared for them before they showed signs of it:

> *Our long-term residents with dementia had progressed with the disease in our care. I found this easier because I knew them.*

However, she also indicated that this was only if they were not physically fit: this was the participant who had indicated, in answer to 'What is your experience of dementia?' that fit and active residents with dementia 'exhausted' her and the other residents.

Real satisfaction in caring of people with dementia was shown by five participants. They described their feelings as 'a feeling of great achievement when a resident responds or relearns basic skills'; 'mostly fulfilled'; 'feel more confident and love looking after people with dementia'; 'very challenging and rewarding now'; and 'I get great satisfaction'. However, four of them felt that they had learnt personal skills over a period of time and possibly by trial and error. One said:

> *I have come to feel more confident and love looking after people with dementia.*

This indicates a sense of 'cracking' the care of people with dementia.

These participants had very different personal recipes for success. They included a number of years of practical experience combined with education; giving a high standard in the package of care to residents that gave them a good quality of life; knowing that it is necessary to give people with dementia reassurance and understanding and being someone who can listen to them; and give help and support to the person and their family as individuals. This last participant also included that one can only do this by looking at oneself and that not everyone is suited to this kind of work. These comments came from four participants who had been caring for people with dementia for between three years and 13 years, therefore length of time did not seem to be necessary in order to find a personal remedy and achieve personal satisfaction. However, achieving a personal strategy did seem to be necessary in order to gain satisfaction.

Why did you come on the course?

The third question on the precourse information sheet asked 'Why did you come on the course?' Fourteen participants said they wished to gain knowledge or more knowledge about dementia or to understand it. Ten of them qualified this by saying that this was for the benefit of the people with dementia; to 'improve my approach to their care' or 'to understand how best to help the clients cope with dementia' were typical comments. One of these participants qualified this further by saying that she wanted to:

> help the residents in the dementia unit to lead fuller and more satisfying lives.

Two of the most experienced participants (one said she had 19 years of experience, the other 13 years) wanted to update their knowledge and learn about new skills and new areas. The latter said:

> There seems to be more available today – many different people/groups are looking at dementia. Today's thoughts will be more research based too. It may also endorse the way in which I look after p.w.d.

This participant clearly has considerable up-to-date knowledge of health care generally in order to know about research-based care. However, she is looking to measure her skills against those of other people and against research, thus showing a very outward-looking approach to care. She is likely to be someone who reads about and discusses care with other people. By doing this, she is probably already developing her own methods of life-long learning. However, what is interesting about her responses to all the questions is that she does not mention that this knowledge will be of benefit to her staff or the relatives but only to her clients with dementia. As a manager of an organisation, I wonder if life-long learning for her indicates purely self-development, rather than sharing this with others. This could be one of the problems with life-long learning in a culture where we are all individuals.

As well as gaining knowledge for themselves, four participants wanted to take this knowledge back to their organisation for the benefit of other staff, one of these also mentioning the gain for the families (organisation D).

A further participant had very specific needs – to learn more about dementia as her number of respite admissions was increasing and these were in the later stage of dementia. This may well account for her previous comment about the disruption to the home caused by one very active lady in the later stages of dementia who exhausted them all. This participant also referred to the Community Care Act which meant her home did not receive admissions to long-term care so readily as in the past, as older people now remained in their own homes for longer. She also knew that special training was needed in care for people with dementia in order for the home to be classed as a specialist dementia unit. In the following question this participant said she wished to have her home registered as a dementia unit.

One participant said she was 'asked by my manager' and this formed her only stated reason for wanting to come on the course. This was despite her saying she felt frustrated and sad and wondered if there was any other way of dealing with situations. I therefore assumed that she did not feel education was a particularly valid method of gaining further knowledge in order to deal with practical problems.

What do you hope to be able to do at the end of the course that you could not do before it?

The last question on the precourse information sheet asked participants 'What do you hope to be able to do at the end of this course that you could not do before it?' There were two categories of response to this question: one indicated self-improvement; the other improvement for others, including staff and relatives. In self-improvement, participants hoped for a number of different personal outcomes including:

- to be able to understand people with dementia better and how to help them;
- to understand the different types of dementia in order to be able to help clients in an individual way;
- to have something better to offer residents with dementia;
- to plan better care;
- to work better with clients;

- to increase personal confidence and therefore success in caring for people with dementia;
- to be more efficient in care for people with dementia.

The last remark indicates the severe pressure put on the whole organisation by a single resident with dementia. The penultimate comment also indicates a similar theme; although this participant had 13 years experience in care of people with dementia she shows how being unable to influence the person with dementia causes her a severe lack of confidence in her own abilities. Thus, as a manager of the home, she feels unable to teach or show her staff how to care, so increasing her loss of confidence. She shows this clearly in her final comment:

I hope to have even more understanding of the disease/illness and how p.w.d. think and behave.

Therefore, although she showed tendencies to life-long learning in response to the previous question, she has not been able to find out how to overcome the problems of care for some people with dementia in her organisation. Until she has found this, it seems that she will be unable to consider how she might use the knowledge and skills to the benefit of others. The sense of loss of confidence in one's own abilities was echoed by another participant from the same home who said she wanted to be able to be 'more positive about the disease'. A further participant also had difficulty in getting through to her clients with dementia as she said she hoped to be able to 'make myself better understood'. Participants with considerable experience and confidence in their abilities to care for older people, when faced with people with dementia, have their confidence undermined so that it evaporates like the morning dew, leaving them very vulnerable and uncertain and threatening their self-esteem.

Two participants expressed a single hope – to understand dementia care mapping.

In the set of responses that indicated improvement for others, five participants indicated that they hoped to pass the information onto other, more junior care staff or to share the learning with other fellow workers. Passing information to more junior staff indicates that the participant puts herself in a hierarchy in her organisation, whereas to share learning with other fellow workers shows more of a system of equality, despite the participant's position in the organisation. A further comment, from an owner/manager of an organisation (organisation A), shows that apart from updating herself, she hopes to:

ensure other participants on this course from the home have support in teaching junior staff.

This comment shows considerable managerial style in ensuring the information is not simply learnt by herself and her more senior staff, but that she intends that the knowledge will be used by other staff in the home. It also shows a hierarchical system of staff.

A further participant, rather than indicating other staff for which he had responsibility, indicated that he wished to use the knowledge to 'bash' the committee of the home:

To be able to influence the policy of the home's committee.

This participant also wished to be able to 'work more efficiently with doctors and other specialists', indicating that more equality with these groups was an expectation.

A further comment on this aspect was that to further one participant's aims for her home to be registered as a dementia unit, she needed to have her staff trained in dementia care. This was evidently her prime aim in attending – to persuade the quality assurance unit to register her home as a specialist unit for dementia, as a way of increasing her bed occupancy.

Those who hoped to use their knowledge for the benefit of the families of older people with dementia (three participants) indicated that they wanted to help the families to 'come to terms with their relative's decline'. One participant did not complete this question; she had over eight years experience in a specialist unit for people with dementia and indicated, in response to the previous question, that she wanted to pass on her knowledge to other staff in the home.

In summary, before any teaching began the participants had a considerable variation in their length of time and experience in caring for people with dementia. This experience was often associated with courses and contact with professionals working in the field. Some nurses felt that a psychiatric training is of benefit. However, caring for a relative with dementia was seen as a less valid experience than caring in a professional capacity. The knowledge of the stages of dementia, its prevalence and how to care was very varied and did not depend on the length of time participants had worked with people with dementia. Some participants saw their caring role being for relatives as well as for the clients themselves. A few participants saw the disruption caused to their organisation by active people with dementia as unacceptable.

Participants felt a sense of frustration and satisfaction in equal measures in caring for people with dementia. Both of these feelings could be quite extreme and did not depend on the length of time the participant had been caring for people with dementia. Some participants also indicated the sense of physical exhaustion, depending on the organisation of the home and their role in it, and one participant indicated that a previous course had not given the necessary skills or understanding for this type of caring. Finding care for people with dementia satisfying and rewarding was said to depend on knowing them over a long period of time and also developing a personal remedy for success.

Almost all participants wanted to learn more about dementia, to gain knowledge and understanding or to update their knowledge in order to improve their care. Most of them also wanted to pass this on to their staff; however, one participant wanted to use it as a strategy for increasing the organisation's bed occupancy, while another wanted it as a weapon to persuade the committee. By the end of the programme participants hoped to have improved themselves and also to be able to improve the lot of others, including relatives. Self-improvement included quite specific aims as well as more general aims such as improving self-confidence which had been sapped by not knowing how to provide adequate care for some of their clients. Those who hoped to be able to improve the knowledge of others in their organisation showed varying levels of bureaucracy.

THE TAUGHT PART OF THE COURSE

The remainder of this chapter will discuss the taught part of the programme. The sessions in the individual organisations to promote self-directed learning will form the content of the next chapter.

Following completion of the precourse information sheets, a brief introduction by me and each participant introducing themselves, I outlined my understanding of the agreement I had reached with each organisation individually on the nature and content of the programme. Everyone agreed that there should be two days of teaching, with three days in between each (two of which would be a weekend), in which participants would read material relating to the previous day's teaching. These two days of teaching would be followed by eight hours in each organisation working with participants to look at ways of trying to understand clients with dementia who were causing particular difficulty. I emphasised that the participants themselves were the experts in caring for people with dementia but that I could suggest ways of obtaining knowledge about their particular clients' needs from a number of sources and help them to try out this knowledge to see if and how it worked. This was generally agreed by all.

At the start of the programme I indicated that the approach to dementia roughly fell into two main areas:

- one area explained dementia by referring to the degenerative processes in the brain and the associated behaviour problems that this caused;
- the second area acknowledged this but felt that by far the most important influence on the person's behaviour was the social processes involved in everyday care for the person with dementia.

It seemed appropriate to make this clear distinction by organising the first of the two days of teaching around the first area and the second day around the second area. In line with good teaching practice, the days were participative and we broke after each hour in order to relax and socialise for a few minutes.

The first day was organised around the well-known book *Understanding Dementia* by Alan Jacques (1988) which takes a biological approach to dementia and discusses the physiological processes in degeneration of nerves and the associated behaviour changes that this causes. I also introduced some material from Chapman & Fraser (1997). At the end of the day I gave each participant some reading on this approach. We agreed to meet three days later for the second of the two days.

The following day I received a telephone call from a participant in organisation E to say that she knew all that we had covered the previous day and thought the course was going to be on dementia care mapping. I explained that this would form the content of the second day. However, I was worried that we appeared to have a lack of understanding, despite what I felt to be my careful initial negotiations. She seemed appeased at my explanation and all three participants from this organisation attended the second day.

At the beginning of the second day of teaching, I emphasised that the day's approach would be quite different from that of the previous day. It would not undermine what had been learnt on the first day but was an approach to dementia which came from a different standpoint – that of the social sciences. For this day, I structured teaching around ideas of personhood (Graham, 1992) and the work of Kitwood (1990a, b, 1991–2, 1992) and Kitwood & Bredin (1991). Following this day I also gave reading in the area.

Both days went well, apart from the intervening telephone call, which appeared to be fully resolved after the second day of teaching. Also, each organisation was very keen to use their eight hours and wanted to arrange dates for these as soon as the teaching was finished. I did not use a post-teaching questionnaire, as I felt feedback would be automatically given during the sessions with the individual organisations.

SUMMARY

In this chapter I have shown how knowledge about dementia was negotiated with a number of organisations in order to promote life-long learning in their senior staff. In order that everyone had a background knowledge of dementia, we agreed that it would be better to have two initial days of teaching, which would be followed up by consideration with the participants of their individual clients with dementia in their own organisation. These follow-up sessions would enable participants to use their knowledge and to develop more particular knowledge in care for their clients with dementia. By looking for knowledge that we agreed was needed and by using it with individual clients, we would not only find out what worked but the areas in which there was no knowledge available. The follow-up sessions with the individual organisations and their approach to this part of the programme, which was specifically designed to aid their individual self-directed learning, are the subject of the next chapter.

REFERENCES

Burgess, R.G. (1991) *In the Field: An Introduction to Field Research*. Routledge, London.

Chapman, A. and Fraser, M. (1997) *Dementia: A Self-Study Pack*. University of Stirling, Dementia Services Development Centre, Stirling.

Graham, G. (1992) *Philosophy of Mind: An Introduction*. Blackwell, Oxford, pp. 154–177.

Jacques, A. (1988) *Understanding Dementia*. Churchill Livingstone, Edinburgh.

Kitwood, T. (1990a) The dialectics of dementia: with particular reference to Alzheimer's disease. *Ageing and Society*, **10**, 177–196.

Kitwood, T. (1990b) Towards a psychology of moral life. In: *Concern for Others: A New Psychology of Conscience and Morality*, (ed. T. Kitwood), Routledge, London, pp. 39–68.

Kitwood, T. (1991–2) Evaluating quality of care in formal settings. *Alzheimer's Disease Society Newsletter*, Dec/Jan, 5.

Kitwood, T. (1992) Quality assurance in dementia care. *Geriatric Medicine*, September, 34–38.

Kitwood, T. and Bredin, K. (1992) *Person to Person*, 2nd edn. Gala Centre Publications, Loughton, Essex.

Lofland, J. and Lofland, L. (1995) *Analysing Social Settings: A Guide to Qualitative Observation and Analysis*. Wadsworth, Belmont, California.

Watson, R. (1997) Ethnomethodology and textual analysis. In: *Qualitative Research: Theory, Method and Practice*, (ed. D. Silverman) Sage, London, pp. 80–98.

6 THE PLEASURE – AND A LITTLE PAIN – OF SELF-DIRECTED LEARNING

In this chapter I will discuss the different organisations' and individuals' responses to the promotion of self-directed learning. I will also consider this against the individuals' precourse information sheets to show how plans were set and needs were developed. I will discuss self-directed learning according to each participating organisation, as the individuals in each organisation generally worked together in this part of the programme.

The initial two-day course on dementia was held during May. The follow-up eight hours for each organisation took place from mid-May until September of the same year. In each organisation I emphasised that these sessions were to help participants to understand and develop ways of caring for individual clients, possibly those that were causing staff the most difficulty.

In order to save the reader having to refer back to the previous chapter to find reference to the organisations, I will repeat their brief details at the beginning of each relevant section below.

ORGANISATION A

Organisation A was a long-term private residential home for care of older people. It had recently opened a new wing. Its care staff were undergoing VQs at levels II and III. Its owner, who was also heavily involved in running the home, participated with two of her senior care staff.

I met with participants in this home four times during June to September. All three participants were very eager to discuss their clients with dementia and the particular difficulties they posed. There were two clients that were causing them particular difficulty: one (AC) had occasions when she would not co-operate with carers in such activities as putting her false teeth in and taking them out; she also ate with her fingers and took exception to some of the other residents and was verbally abusive to them. The second resident (AM) had more severe problems, showing great fear particularly when taken to the toilet and being undressed to use the toilet, as well as when going to bed; she would shout and swear and dig her nails into the carers on many occasions so that carers began to dread taking her to the toilet or performing personal hygiene activities. There was also often a struggle to put her false teeth in and to take them out. In discussion, we felt that she was probably interpreting being undressed and being taken to the toilet as physical assault and so was protesting loudly, although in between times was quiet and peaceful; she would also occasionally throw drinks at people. This, according to the participants, appeared to form a pattern, as she was said to have shown signs of paranoia before becoming a resident in the home.

The three participants from this organisation said, in the precourse information sheet, that they wanted a better understanding of dementia so as to help their clients to cope with dementia and improve their life.

We discussed the use of life story books (Murphy, 1994) and, through the development of these, how participants could help staff to understand the clients' behaviour better. Participants wanted to develop this at a later stage but it was not a priority while the existing problems were so severe.

In discussing AM's apparent likes, we considered how she would sit and hold someone's hand; we therefore felt her distress could be seen as a lack of security. As it was impractical for staff to sit and hold her hand for any length of time, I was asked to find some information that might help us to understand her response better and we could then see how the information worked. In searching for material from a local resource I came across doll therapy (Godfrey, 1994) which promoted the idea of dolls being a way for people with dementia to achieve feelings of security. On my second visit I took the article with me and discussed it with the participants, who thought it might provide an answer and agreed to try out the ideas. Not only did they want to try it out but they also volunteered to keep diaries of how AM responded. I was delighted that they wished to do so but felt somewhat guilty at the extra work involved, but they were very keen to document their progress.

On my third visit, three weeks later, the participants told me of the partial success of doll therapy with AM and handed me the sheets from the diaries, completed daily by different carers. On this occasion the owner/manager did not join us. However, it was evident that other staff in the home had also been involved in writing the diaries. Diary entries on both clients continued daily from the middle of June until the end of July. The diary entries are analysed below, again according to Watson (1997). So that readers may check the accuracy of my interpretations, I include the complete diary entries as Appendix 1.

It is evident from the diary entries that carers see certain areas as central to AM, for example mood. Almost every entry mentions this:

13.6.96
Today A's mood was very good. She responded well to anything that was said to her.
IK

AM is referred to as agitated when her mood is poor. Therefore the general description of AM seems to be agreed between all the staff, including the participants on the programme. There are also some very perceptive reasons for why her mood might not be good, including that she is constipated:

20.6.96
A in great fettle today. Has eaten and drunk well. She has been a delight to look after. I think her cheerfulness is due to a bowel movement, as when she is constipated, she is very tetchy.
IK

This could well lead to the carer taking particular note of bowel movements and maybe taking some action when they have been absent for a few days. Also noticed by a carer is mood changes in relation to the carer's personal appearance:

17.6.96
Have noticed A's mood changes when I put my hair up; she never recognises me. When I had my hair down A was laughing and talking again.
JL

These types of observations might result in the carer adopting certain sorts of behaviour, such as wearing her hair down to help the client recognise her. Both the comments on bowel movements and how hair is worn are made by two carers who did not attend the programme. As the daily dairies were used by a large number of carers, as well as the two senior carers who attended the programme, the diaries were seen by everyone in the organisation and were not merely written for me to read. Therefore forming theories about behaviour and testing them out appears to be an acceptable way of behaving in this organisation. On this evidence it could well be that this organisation is encouraging movement towards life-long learning by encouraging its staff to adopt this approach. However, less good is that this theorising appears to be occurring in individuals and the areas observed and commented upon do not seem to be those that other carers also mention, for example, constipation being associated with mood changes is only mentioned by IK. Therefore, on this evidence, staff are tending to formulate their own theories but are acting as individuals, rather than sharing them to make an impact on others, or are sharing their theorising with others but are having their ideas rejected. However, the systems used by this organisation to encourage sharing of ideas between staff are not known.

Client AC is not seen in the same way as AM, as mood is mentioned on only one entry. She is described as being restless or calm:

5.7.96
On getting A ready for bed she was very restless going back and forwards from the toilet to the door; she did not want her clothes taken off because she was very cold; once ready for bed, sat her in the lounge where she continued to get up and down asking for her sister; put on some music for her and she seems to have settled down a bit.
AS

These ways of seeing AC seem to be similar in most of the carers who wrote in the diary. Diary entries on AC and AM show evidence that staff of all grades recognise individual differences between clients. Therefore staff in this organisation are not only able to theorise about their work and change their practice accordingly, but are able to act on individual differences that they recognise in their clients.

In relation to the success of doll therapy, these two processes (forming theories about behaviour and recognising individual differences) are seen. There were a number of entries showing how the teddy bear given to AM had been responded to:

24.6.96
A was in a brilliant mood today, we gave her one of O's teddy's to see how she reacted and the reaction was great and A thought it was lovely.
MM

This shows staff trying out the teddy to see if it had the effects described in the article. As the doll was seen to be a success, it was tried again in other circumstances when AM's mood was seen to be poor:

3.7.96
A had a bath this morning, upset when getting hair washed and weighed. Given her teddy which helped to calm her while I was drying her and her hair and this helped a lot.
MC

and

28.7.96
When preparing for bed got a little aggressive. Gave her one of her teddies and sat with her talking and playing with teddy until she was laughing again and then finished getting her ready for bed with no trouble.
MC

This again shows evidence of testing theories in a practical sense in different situations by using the information from other sources to see how it worked. However, the staff who wrote about the use of doll therapy were the participants who attended the two-day course; therefore in the other entries where the client shows aggressive behaviour no attempts to use the doll are seen. Participants on the programme carried on using doll therapy, once they saw it was successful, and it continued to have success in calming the client, so making it easier for them to provide care. However, according to the senior care staff who participated in the programme it did not always provide the required change in the client's mood and one of the diary entries shows this:

7.7.96
A very tired when being put to bed and was very agitated. Tried giving her
the teddy but this did not help.
MC

In the same way that other carers formed theories and tested them in practice, as shown in the two quotations above about the effects on the client of the carer wearing hair in a particular way and of the client being constipated, the participants on the programme (MC and MM) had tested out new information with some success. However, they too had either failed to get the message across to the other staff or had not shared the information with them as there is no reference by any other carer to the use of a doll.

On this third visit at the beginning of July I was asked to go with the two senior carers to see AM and she was holding her teddy close to her; I was told she always had it with her. However, the significance of this seemed to have eluded the rest of the staff, according to the diary entries.

Client AC was also introduced to dolls by one of the participants on the programme, but did not seem to be interested in them:

16.7.96
A woke up at 8.45 and seemed more settled, was shown a lot of soft toys to
ask if she would like one but did not want one.
MC

The two senior care staff said they thought the reason for the success of the doll with one client and not the other was that AM had been a mother and had loved her children, whereas AC had never married and therefore possibly had not had the close contact with toys and small, warm and cuddly objects. Therefore, these staff were able to bring the background of the client into the evaluations of success.

At the end of the third visit the two participants said they would like to continue to use doll therapy as it seemed to be making a marked improvement, rather than moving onto other areas. They also felt that in making changes to caring, it was important to establish a change with all carers before moving onto something else. On the fourth visit in the middle of September doll therapy was still being practised and evaluated by the two participants as making a significant difference to AM, although AC had continued to show no interest. However, there was no sign from the diaries that the ideas or practice had percolated down to the rest of the staff.

Summary of organisation A's response

This organisation showed that some of its staff were evidently ripe for self-directed learning. The two participants on the programme were keen to try out new ideas; they were able to identify the areas in which they most needed help and to keep diaries of how new information helped them to understand their clients better. They were also able to persuade other staff to keep the diary. They were able to use information to alleviate problems and to evaluate its effectiveness. Their ability to promote the use of critical reflection on practice in other staff was evidenced by the fact that all staff caring for the two residents used diaries of their practice. However, the two participants (MC and MM, see Appendix 1) failed to promote new areas of practice for use by the rest of the staff and so change their practice in spite of having evaluated the changes as being beneficial for one of their clients. Therefore the owner/manager's claim in her precourse information sheet that she would 'ensure other participants on this course from the home have my support in teaching junior staff' was not seen to occur in the instance of doll therapy. However, participants showed a very mature approach to the speed at which new information could be assimilated into the organisation in order to make a real difference to practice but even six weeks after they claimed to be using new ideas themselves with success, the ideas had not been taken up by other staff.

However, other staff were evidently encouraged to be observant of the behaviour of their clients and to form theories about what was making a difference to their behaviour, so that they could also learn from their experience. However, these other staff appeared equally unable to persuade others to accept their ideas and so remained isolated with their individual theories. This organisation therefore tended to encourage staff to critically evaluate clients' behaviour, but failed to capitalise on this to the benefit of everyone. Thus, they would probably eventually stifle individual creativity so that the organisation as a whole would not be able to change rapidly.

As an organisation they also lacked knowledge of where information to help them to understand and solve problems could be found, as well as the ability to find this information for themselves. This also appeared to be a major problem for all but one of the other organisations on the programme. This is possibly one of the main constraints to small businesses becoming learning organisations.

ORGANISATION B

Organisation B was a voluntary organisation providing domiciliary support for all age groups. They had a part-time trainer who was assessing VQs to level II. It was their trainer who participated.

I visited the participant in this organisation on three occasions. Her needs were to have something that would not only be useful and interesting but also as a form of therapy for both the client and the carer. As she explained to me, it is often difficult for a carer to be with a client in their own home for long periods of time (up to six hours at a stretch). They both often ran out of conversation after a short period of time, particularly if they had been together recently. If they had something useful and interesting to do, this would make the time enjoyable for both parties as well as providing a sense of purpose. As this participant had a good understanding of dementia from her previous two years of training and four years working with clients with dementia in a domiciliary setting, she was aware of some of the areas we might consider and had used them in long-term care settings. From this first meeting we agreed it would be useful to consider reality orientation (RO) and reminiscence therapy (RT) in relation to their use in the domiciliary setting. We both agreed to find out more about this and to meet again the following week.

On my second visit the participant had located two sources of objects that might be used in RT: a sweet shop selling sweets similar to those produced at the beginning of the century, such as pear drops, and a museum that lent articles in common use at the beginning of the century, such as small enamel jugs and baking shapes. I produced articles on how RO and RT could be conducted (Parker & Somers, 1983; Archibald, 1991; Phair & Elsey, 1990; Osborn, 1989). Between the objects and the articles, the participant was able to organise both RO and RT experiences for her clients and to help her carers to do this.

We discussed how a programme for one or two care assistants could be created – the participant identified one or two clients that she could visit with the care assistants in order to discuss this and set it up. She wanted to establish her ideas and practise them with a few selected clients in order to evaluate the results before making them more widely available. We agreed to meet the following week to consider progress.

On the third visit a very different story emerged. The organisation had had its funding cut due to local government reorganisation, which the participant interpreted as her job being under threat. It was therefore not possible to discuss any of the areas we had previously considered, due to the participant's level of agitation. As she was the only trainer in the organisation she evidently felt somewhat isolated with her concerns. I was therefore put in the position of counsellor while she discussed her worries and problems with her job. Shortly after this visit she left her job to take up work with a different organisation.

Summary of Organisation B's response

The single participant from organisation B had a good record of training in care for people with dementia and also of experience in caring for such people, particularly in a domiciliary setting. Her greatest need appeared to be someone with whom to discuss approaches to teaching and learning, due to her isolated position in the organisation. She had evident skills of identifying her needs, being able to locate practical resources and plan how to use them in combination with carers and clients. The organisation in which she worked supported her approach and she did not appear to have the same constraints on finding appropriate resources to develop her knowledge as did the participants in organisation A. Therefore this organisation was possibly more able to develop life-long learning provided it was able to achieve financial stability.

However, events overtook the participant before she could put her ideas into practice and could evaluate them. As we can see from Chapter 1, these kinds of crises in voluntary organisations are not unknown. Changing conditions of employment for staff and the resulting loss of morale are also not unknown in research when trying to make changes in an organisation, as Baron, Gilloran & Schad (1995) found when trying to set up an audit system with community mental handicap nurses.

ORGANISATION C

Organisation C was a long-term private residential home for older people; they had just opened a new, purpose-built wing for people with dementia. They were involved in training their care staff to VQ level II. Two of their senior care staff involved in the new dementia wing partici-pated, one of whom had recently completed a level III VQ.

I visited this organisation four times during May and June. Because of the newness of the unit, the needs of the staff were greater than those of some of the other organisations. One particular resident, whose husband had died eight weeks beforehand, had moved into the unit shortly afterwards. The staff wanted to help her to grieve and also to provide support for her family. They had also found that when one of their residents became emotional, all the other residents became emotional too; they likened this to mass hysteria, as one person's behaviour set off the others. Participants had also noticed that clients became more prone to wander and cause disruption at a certain time in the afternoon; this had happened regularly. Participants also wanted to know about dementia care mapping and to develop more appropriate care plans for people with dementia. There were therefore a number of areas which needed to be considered.

I agreed to find information on all these areas and to meet the two members of staff again the following week. In the intervening week I was able to find information on the grieving process (Johnson, Morton & Knox, 1992; Lloyd, 1992), on the Sundown Syndrome (Wallace, 1994; Gerdner & Buckwalter, 1994) and on dementia care mapping (Kitwood & Bredin, 1992; 1994; Barnett, 1995). As there were so many areas to cover, I summarised some of them, for example the grieving process, and dementia care mapping, in order not to overburden the participants. Summarising the topic combined with discussion with the participants as well as giving them the articles appeared to work well.

On meeting with the participants the following week I was again struck by the enormous sense of tension in the staff. One of the partici-pants found particular difficulty sitting down to discuss the areas in which she had expressed problems; in the precourse information sheet, she had stated a need to 'deal with certain situations better' as well as to gain more experience and knowledge about dementia. However, the other participant was able to do so and the two of us fully discussed the three areas and I left her with the information I had collected and prepared. However, there were also other areas she wished to know more about; these included borrowing a video on the effects of nerve degeneration on behaviour, which they wished to use for staff training, and help with understanding and knowing how to respond to sexual behaviour between two of the residents. I said I would follow up these two areas and we agreed to meet again in two weeks.

On the following visit I took with me the video *Brain and Behaviour* (Alzheimer's Association of Australia, 1995) and *Sexuality and Dementia* (Dementia Services Development Centre, 1996). At this visit, one participant discussed with me how the client who had been bereaved was gradually becoming less distressed and how the family was also becoming more involved and able to support her. Although they were still experiencing the disruption by all their clients at certain times of day, they now knew what to expect and therefore had rearranged their shift patterns for more staff to be on duty at this time. They were also writing a guide for all staff on the unit which included some advanced graphics, in which many of the articles we had discussed had been used. I was asked to comment on this. Understandably, with this level of development, they had not been able to sufficiently concentrate on dementia care mapping to make any headway.

At this third meeting they also wanted information on holding staff meetings as a way of handling the stress in the unit; it was felt that this might provide a release of tension. They also wanted information on assessment of residents before they came into the unit. The information I found for them was taken from Gregory (1991), Wright (1990) and *Carenap D* (Fife Health Care, n.d.), which is used by assessment teams. We again discussed these fully at the last meeting I had with them.

At the last meeting we reviewed what they had achieved. They had virtually completed the handbook for carers, which looked very impressive. They had held their first staff meeting and encouraged everyone to comment on their experience of working in the unit and asked for suggestions for improvement. This was said to have been productive and was felt to be needed as a forum, as every member of staff had attended, including those on a day off.

Staff had come to terms with clients being distressed together and the change in shift patterns meant there were now more carers around to supervise these occasions. They had also worked through a problem of two of the residents (one male and one female) going into each other's bedrooms for long periods of time and had warned the staff not to go into the rooms during these periods. They had also been able to discuss the situation with the two people concerned and with their close family, who gave their approval. Although this had given staff considerable moral dilemmas, they had taken the mature approach that if the residents themselves understood and both equally agreed with what they were doing and the nearest relatives had given their approval, then staff should not attempt to stop the activity.

However, despite the considerable achievements of this organisation, the stress levels appeared to remain high. They were also not able to devote sufficient time to using the information on dementia care mapping, but intended to do so.

Summary of organisation C's response

The needs of organisation C were considerable due to the unit having recently opened, with new clients and new staff; everyone needed to achieve harmony in their new surroundings. It was therefore a period of considerable change and adaptation in which everyone was involved and tension was evident. Although the senior carer was very energetic and enthusiastic and was able to achieve a great deal in a very short space of time, the other participant on the programme showed signs of severe stress and left the organisation shortly after the follow-up sessions were complete. With hindsight I could have advised that a slower pace of assimilating information and trying it out might have been beneficial; however, the amount of new knowledge needed was agreed between myself and the senior participant and was in line with their stated needs. However, the depth to which the information was developed and the changes required among all the staff were likely to lead to stress.

In relation to life-long learning in this organisation, the senior participant showed considerable ability to identify her needs and to use the resulting information for the rest of the staff. This was particularly the case in the production of the handbook for staff. However, she relied on me to obtain the information, although she possibly had the ability to find it for herself, given the time to do so. It therefore appeared that this organisation promoted self-development in its staff and expected them to learn the necessary skills, but possibly wanted this at too fast a pace, particularly initially, for everyone. Possibly with a few months of 'bedding down', they will be able to achieve real life-long learning.

ORGANISATION D

Organisation D was a long-term care residential home. They were part of a consortium to assess VQs but progress had been slow. Three of their senior care staff participated, one of whom was the hands-on manager of the home.

I visited this organisation three times from May to July. Discussion with two of their participants (the third was not available), revealed that they did not have problems with any particular client but needed more general information on care for people with dementia. This organisation wished to become registered as a dementia unit. We discussed the more popular areas that had been developed recently, such as life story books, reminiscence therapy and reality orientation. They requested information on life story books (Murphy, 1994) and reminiscence therapy (Osborn, 1989; Phair & Elsey, 1990), which I took to them the following week. They also wanted to visit the specialist organisation for dementia (organisation E) which was arranged in July.

On this second visit only one of the participants was available. The office was occupied, so we made ourselves at home in the kitchen, standing up against the work surfaces. We fully discussed the life story book approach and how it could work, we also discussed how reminiscence therapy could work and that it was possible to borrow items from a local library to help. I left the material with the participant and arranged a third visit for the following week.

Before the next visit I was telephoned to change the date as everyone was on holiday. A further date was set for the following two weeks. On arrival on the planned day nobody was available as the senior participant was visiting the local hospital. I waited for a short while for her return. On her return she said that no progress had been made with the material I had left and that really they had attended the course for the certificate at the end and therefore did not want any more visits.

Summary of organisation D's response

Organisation D appeared, from the precourse information sheets, to have considerable needs for dementia care education, as they wanted to be recognised as a dementia unit to increase their bed occupancy. However, they seemed unable to organise themselves sufficiently to benefit from training directly related to their clients. This was consistent with the slow progress of VQs in the organisation. It could therefore be assumed that their approach to life-long learning was very much in its infancy and that a real culture change would have to occur before they could benefit from such a development.

ORGANISATION E

Organisation E was a purpose-built long-term church home for people with dementia. They had a full-time trainer as part of their staff and an extensive training programme for staff and relatives. The full-time trainer and two senior care staff participated. I did not know this home and its participants before the programme started.

I visited this organisation on three occasions from May to August. Their expressed needs throughout the programme had been to learn more about dementia care mapping (DCM) and this was reinforced at the first meeting. They also wanted a copy of the video *Brain and Behaviour* (Alzheimer's Association of Australia, 1995) to show to their relatives group to help them understand the process of dementia. They wanted copies of the videos on dementia available at the local centre and said they would welcome visits from other participants on the programme.

On my second visit I had selected articles that I thought would be most helpful in understanding DCM (Kitwood & Bredin, 1992, 1994; Barnett, 1995). From these I summarised the essentials of DCM and devised charts that would help us to try it out, although stressing that this was a summary of the articles and did not constitute a course on DCM, the copyright for which is held by the University of Bradford. The participants were very enthusiastic to try it out and we discussed in detail how they might do so and how to set up periods of observation. I stressed that setting up observation was important, including:

- how observation was tiring so frequent breaks would be needed in order not to become exhausted by the experience and so numbed to the detail of what was being observed;
- that it was important to gain agreement of those being observed in order that they would not find the process intrusive.

We also discussed feelings of isolation and stress that have been noted by observers (Lofland & Lofland, 1995; Spradley, 1979). The staff organised appropriate times when observation would occur and who should do it. They said this type of participation was not new to the organisation as on one occasion, to get a 'feel' for what it was like to be a client, one of their senior staff had spent the day being a client and had gained some very useful experience which had led to changes in practice.

On my third visit two of the participants had conducted three periods of observation and were immensely enthusiastic about their findings. Not only had they completed the charts I had prepared, but one participant had written copious notes on her observations over two period of 15 minutes each on separate days. On the first day that observation was conducted, she noted the following in relation to Mrs F at breakfast time, while she was also observing two other clients:

1. *(Can be variable at mealtimes. Particularly vague in the morning and*
2. *needs lots of encouragement to eat and drink. Also directives re use of*
3. *cutlery.)*
4. *Had 1/1 with J who was chatting to her giving her eye to eye contact and*
5. *encouraging her to eat and drink. Succeeded. Offered and took another*
6. *piece of toast and was left.*
7. *Vague – looking at toast on plate.*
8. *J noted same and sought to give encouragement.*
9. *Left/still vague/toast on plate/uncut 5 minutes.*
10. *S noted this – sat and gave eye to eye contact – encouraging to drink tea*
11. *– succeeded.*
12. *Cut piece of toast and sought to encourage her to eat same – put piece in*
13. *hand – v. vague unable to coordinate.*
14. *Offered more assistance. Refused.*

Lines 1, 2 and 3 show the participant had a good knowledge of the client and the particular help she needs at this time of day. She not only showed a knowledge of the client but also the differences that she shows according to the time of day. The participant has also clearly positioned herself where she can see the faces of the client and the carers well in order to gauge their responses. Lines 4, 5 and 6 show the strategies used by a carer to help Mrs F to eat and what happens (line 7) when she is left to her own devices. However, the participant also observes that the carer is attentive (line 8) but that this is not necessarily successful (line 9); the phrase 'sought to give encouragement' implies that the carer did all the right things, but that she did not succeed in her aim, as line 9 shows. However, lines 10 and 11 show that another carer is also attentive to the client's needs and, with good eye contact and talking with her, succeeded in persuading the client to eat and drink. However, lines 12–14 indicate that this too was unsuccessful at a second attempt. This series of activities between the two carers and the client was judged favourably by the participant, who also discussed her reaction to observing breakfast for this client which reinforced her favourable view of both carers.

On her second period of observation the participant had evidently gained confidence in the skills needed, as she was able to include the time of events. She again observed for 15 minutes and observed three clients. However, this time she was more critical of how one of the clients was treated:

1. *4.15 Quiet, inactive, watching others from afar.*
2. *4.20 Still watching others but playing with paper hank.*
3. *Repeating some of M's group's conversation. Looking down side of*
4. *chair – playing with paper hank.*
5. *Looking at electric fire.*
6. *Watching others – started to slap/pat leg loudly.*
7. *Looking at hem of skirt.*
8. *4.25 Repeating some of M's group's conversation. Talking to herself.*
9. *Looking up expectantly when V came in. Disappointed when M*
10. *directed her elsewhere. Looking around – put paper on fire.*

During my third visit to this organisation, this was the piece of observation that had excited the participant the most and which she had discussed with her two other colleagues. She said she had no idea the effects that ignoring a client could have, as although this client was only ignored for about 10 minutes, she displayed signs of being distressed, such as shown in lines 3 and 4, 6 and 8–10. The participant found this a very useful experience and vowed to make her observations known to all staff in order for them to be aware that those sitting alone might wish to be drawn into a group. However, the impact on other staff cannot be determined from the notes of the observations and the project did not last long enough for this to be seen.

The participants were immensely pleased with their abilities and said that they, as staff, also needed stimulation in their work. We made plans for how they would share their knowledge and understanding of dementia care mapping with colleagues and relatives along with the social science philosophy upon which it was built.

Summary of organisation E's response

This organisation already had a very good knowledge and many years of practice in care for clients with dementia. Because of their levels of knowledge and skills, they were among the leaders in the field of care for this client group. They therefore needed the stimulation of new areas and to keep themselves updated. Their response to self-directed learning was to identify their very specific training needs, to ask for help in locating them and to be able to use the information in practice. With this help they were well able to use the information and to appreciate the effects it had on staff and residents in evaluating their organisation's care. They were also more prepared for visits by Quality Assurance inspectors as they said they understood more about what observation was aiming to achieve and how the observations would be interpreted. The participants showed a strong inclination to life-long learning; the organisation also possibly showed a similar inclination but this could not be determined directly. However, the participants showed a need for stimulation from outside the organisation and also to know how to locate and use resources to the best possible effects.

ORGANISATION F

Organisation F was a private residential home for care of older people. They said they did not currenty have any residents with dementia but would like to learn about it. They were part of a consortium to undertake VQs but progress had been slow. Two of their senior care staff participated.

As this organisation had always said they did not have any residents with dementia, I visited them only once in May. On this visit they said they would like to keep their options open to contact me in the future but would very much like to visit organisation E to get a 'feel' for care of people with dementia. I set this up for them and talked to them on the telephone about planning their visit in order to get the most out of it. They telephoned me after their visit to let me know how it went and said it was most useful.

Summary of organisation F's response

The participants in this organisation wanted to know more about dementia and also to learn from other providers. They were not in a position to use this knowledge in their organisation but wanted the knowledge and contacts for future potential clients. They have not asked for advice on dementia since, although I have visited the home on other matters. Apart from recognising their needs to know more about a potential area of practice, which spurred them to attend the taught part of the programme, it was not possible to assess their approach, as an organisation, to life-long learning.

ORGANISATION G

Organisation G was a private nursing home for care of older people with a day centre attached. They were involved in VQ training at levels II and III and had made good progress. Their matron, deputy matron and one of the senior care staff who was also a workplace assessor participated.

I made two visits to this organisation where all participants were present and contributed eagerly. They had one client who was causing them considerable problems. She was described as constantly living in the past, when she was a child. Her mood varied from occasionally being happy but mostly sad and agitated. Staff had tried to involve her in a number of activities but her concentration span only lasted for one or two minutes. She was now failing to recognise her son. She was also failing physically but was still wandering; however, because of her physical limitations she was now calling for her mum, rather than being able to go to look for her. Apart from the client herself, this was causing severe disquiet amongst a few of the other residents. We discussed a number of options, including doll therapy as a way of achieving a sense of security and comfort. Participants wanted to try doll therapy to see if it brought any comfort to her. We discussed how they might use doll therapy with this client and I agreed to send the article by Godfrey for them to read.

A further issue on which they wanted advice was the potential for changes in funding of day care as they were aware of an article in a national newspaper on the issue but had not been able to find it. I agreed to look for written material and also to contact those at national level who might have further information. I was able to telephone them with this information.

All the participants volunteered the information that they had found the two days extremely useful and wanted to borrow the video *Brain and Behaviour* to show to staff. They said that one of the effects of the video was to enhance their understanding of the links in dementia between seeing an object and responding to it. The matron said she would now teach the carers that when clients with dementia did not touch their food, in spite of seeing it in front of them and being reminded that it was there, they should not assume the client did not want it and so take it away. She would teach them that by placing the food or cutlery in the client's hands, they would recognise that this was food and would eat it. She said this had been a most useful lesson to her. Both the other participants also said they had found the course most useful, but were unable to say how they would use the material they had learnt, merely that they were now more confident in their approach to people with dementia. This was reflected in their precourse information sheet on which they both wrote that they wanted to know more about dementia but did not have more specific needs.

My second visit six weeks later found that the client who had caused the main problems had died and they had not had a chance to try doll therapy with her. They wanted to know more about dementia care mapping. I agreed to send them the articles used for organisation E and to bring them the other material on my next routine visit.

Summary of organisation G's response

More than anything else, the participants in this organisation appeared to need updating and to be advised of a source from which to gain information, material and equipment. All the participants were clearly able to identify their own needs for information, although one of them was more specific than the other two, but having the time and knowing where to obtain the resources they needed was their main problem. Once they had the information, the matron, at least, was able to decide how useful it was and to show the other staff how to use it. However, the deputy matron and senior carer seemed less able to do this and seemed to respond better to courses rather than to other strategies associated with life-long learning, such as theorising about what may cause problems, knowing where to get information that may help them to understand the problem better and how to assess the effects of changing behaviour. Therefore, it seemed that without the Matron's presence, this organisation may well not be able to continue as a learning organisation as the ability to pose questions about the work, to consider what changes might be needed and to assess the effects of changes was not clearly instilled in the other staff. It would seem that the matron, at the time of the project, had not been able to promote life-long learning as the normal approach to staff development. This follows clearly from her precourse information sheet where she relates to the people with dementia but does not mention staff. In this respect, organisation G shows similar characteristics to organisation A, where there is a shared understanding of individual clients but where employees act as individuals whose observations and theorising about clients makes minimal impression on other staff.

ORGANISATION H

Organisation H was a small church residential home. They were assessing VQs at levels II and III. Their two joint managers participated, one of whom had recently completed a level III VQ.

I visited this home on four occasions from May to July. They had a number of issues with which they wanted help – some were quite novel in relation to the other organisations' needs. On the first visit they mentioned one particular resident who they said 'lacked responsibility'. By this they meant that she would report conversations she had heard to other people, particularly her relatives. They were unsure if she had dementia but one of her relatives did and they wanted to explore her behaviour from this perspective to see if they could obtain any help with managing her care. Apart from talking about other people, she also had eating problems and had gained a considerable amount of weight; they wondered if this was due to 'attention seeking' at mealtimes. She was also very determined. I asked them to give me an example of this, as I was unsure what they meant; they said if she made up her mind to do something, then nothing would stop her. She also appeared to lack concentration and seemed to be unable to cope with too much stimulation: too many people and too much noise made her agitated and she had to move away. She also possibly had a lack of short-term memory. Her relatives had queried with the participants whether it was possible that she had dementia, due to the family history. In this home the number of residents and the emphasis on community living made it difficult not to be included in daily living activities so anyone with habits that annoyed the others was a severe problem for the staff, particularly as all the other residents were fit and active.

Apart from this lady, a further resident had had a number of small strokes and from the taught part of the programme, the two participants realised that he had multi-infarct dementia. They thus gained an understanding of the type of step-wise decline that they might expect for him. The participants also felt he had numerous other health and social problems, including staring in a vacant manner on occasions.

We agreed that it would be most appropriate to consider whether it was likely that their first client had signs of dementia. As her parents had a history of dementia, I was asked to search for evidence that dementia was hereditary. Looking in the local resource, I noted considerable debate in this area, showing that there was some evidence that dementia was inherited and that this was currently being hotly pursued (Hocking & Breitner, 1995). It appeared that vitamin B_{12} deficiency is hereditary and has a possible relationship with dementia (McCaddon & Kelly, 1994). There was also evidence that heredity was implicated in early-onset Alzheimer's type dementia which was linked to chromosomes 14 and 21 (Plassman & Breitner, 1996; Post, 1994; Mullan, 1992). As well as vitamin B_{12} and chromosomal evidence, there was also some evidence in other areas of heredity and dementia but it appeared that the link was unclear (Giacobini, 1995).

On the second visit this information encouraged the participants to want to explore the facilities they should be providing in the home in order to keep clients with dementia and not to have to send them to another organisation (a previous resident with dementia had been trans-ferred to a more specialist home for long-term care). The participants wanted to be able to convince the committee that it was good practice to keep residents, rather than transfer them elsewhere. We therefore considered the structure of the building that was recommended for people with dementia by studying Kelly (1993) and the different recommendations that needed to be adopted in order for the building to achieve the standards. The participants wanted to take this to the home's committee in a bid to persuade them to make the necessary alterations. This was one of the aims of one participant – 'to be able to influence the policy of the home's committee'.

They also wished to know more about the way in which potential residents were assessed for residential care. I therefore discussed *Carenap-D* with them which was used by the inspection team.

Summary of organisation H's response

This home, and the participants from it, evidently had very different needs from the other organisations on the programme. They said they had learnt a great deal from the taught part of the programme and appeared to be able to identify their learning needs in the follow-up time. However, many of their needs appeared to be driven by frustration with their jobs and the problems they appeared to have with the management of their organisation, which they made explicit and for which they were looking for support. They seemed well able to under-stand and discuss the information provided in response to their requests but they did not appear able to use the information in a meaningful way due to the constraints they felt were on their role. They left the organi-sation shortly after the programme ended.

OVERALL CONCLUSIONS

In this part of the programme the participants in each organisation were encouraged to set their own goals and decide which aspects of dementia to pursue according to their needs and the needs of their residents as they saw them. It was clear that participants within each organisation had very different approaches to learning, which either helped or hindered their willingness to be self-directed. However, the main difference was between each organisation's approach to self-directed or life-long learning. The organisation's approach would be likely to influence not only the participants on the programme but also everyone else involved in care.

Organisations fell into four main groups.

- Two organisations were very actively seeking new information (organisations C and E). They were clearly able to identify their needs for knowledge and looked to someone outside the organisation to help them locate the necessary information. Although the participants were able to use the information effectively, (although one participant from organisation C could not do so due to high levels of stress) I could not determine whether the information was effectively taken up by all the staff in the organisation. However, the organisations had considerable energy and enthusiasm for learning and promoted learning in their senior staff.
- Two of the other organisations were also very actively seeking new information (organisations B and H) but their problems with management limited their ability to implement any of the material. All the members of staff who attended the course left shortly after its completion.
- A further two organisations (organisations A and G) expressed their needs for information on dementia. However, their ability to use it was limited to themselves as individuals, as they appeared not to pass the information on to others with whom they worked.
- The last two organisations understood the need for training but did not appear to appreciate how it could be used to make a difference to the care of their residents. They appeared not to have a questioning approach to care and also seemed to be far more involved in getting through the daily work than considering how education and training could allow different options to emerge.

In the final chapter I will make a few recommendations on how self-directed learning can develop in the context of care for older people.

REFERENCES

Alzheimer's Association of Australia (1995) *Brain and Behaviour*. Video

Archibald, C. (1991) *Activities I & II*. University of Stirling, Dementia Services Development Centre, Stirling.

Barnett, E. (1995) A window of insight into quality care. *Journal of Dementia Care*, July/August, 23–26.

Baron, S., Gilloran, A. and Schad, D. (1995) Collaboration in a time of change: blocks to collaboration. *Social Sciences in Health*, **1(4)**, 195–205.

Dementia Services Development Centre (1996) *Sexuality and Dementia: A Guide*. University of Stirling, Stirling.

Fife Health Care. (n.d.) *Carenap-D*. Dementia Needs Assessment Project, Cupar, Fife.

Gerdner, L.A. and Buckwalter, K.C. (1994) Assessment and management of agitation in Alzheimer's patients. *Journal of Gerontological Nursing*, April, 11–19.

Giacobini, E. (1995) The hot summer of Alzheimer genes. *Alzheimer Insights*, **1**, (1), 5–6.

Godfrey, S. (1994) Doll therapy. *Australian Journal on Aging*, 13(1), 46.

Gregory, S. (1991) Stress management for carers. *British Journal of Occupational Therapy*, **54(11)**, 427–429.

Hocking, L.B. and Breitner, J.C.S. (1995) Cumulative risk of Alzheimer-like dementia in relatives of autopsy-confirmed cases of Alzheimer's disease. *Dementia*, **6**, 355–356.

Johnson, M.A., Morton, M.K. and Knox, S.M. (1992) The transition to a nursing home: meeting the family's needs. *Geriatric Nursing*, November/December, 299–302.

Kelly, M. (1993) *Designing for People with Dementia in the Context of the Building Standards*. University of Stirling, Dementia Services Development Centre, Stirling.

Kitwood, T. and Bredin, K. (1992) A new approach to the evaluation of dementia care. *Journal of Advances in Health and Nursing Care*, **1(5)**, 41–60.

Kitwood, T. and Bredin, K. (1994) Charting the course of quality care. *Journal of Dementia Care*, May/June, 22–23.

Lloyd, M. (1992) Tools for many trades: reaffirming the use of grief counselling by health, welfare and pastoral workers. *British Journal of Guidance and Counselling*, **20(2)**, 150–163.

Lofland, J. and Lofland, L. (1995) *Analysing Social Settings: A Guide to Qualitative Observation and Analysis*. Wadsworth, Belmont, California.

McCaddon, A. and Kelly, C.L. (1994) Familial Alzheimer's disease and Vitamin B_{12} deficiency. *Age and Ageing*, **23**, 334–337.

Mullan, M. (1992) Familial Alzheimer's disease: second gene locus located. *British Medical Journal*, **305**, 1108.

Murphy, C. (1994) *It Started with a Sea-shell: Life Story Work and People with Dementia.* University of Stirling, Dementia Services Development Centre, Stirling.

Osborn, C. L. (1989) Reminiscence: when the past eases the present. *Journal of Gerontological Nursing* **15,** (10), 6–11.

Parker, C. and Somers, C. (1983) Reality orientation on a geropsychiatric unit. *Geriatric Nursing,* May/June, 163–165.

Phair, L. and Elsey, I. (1990) Sharing memories. *Nursing Times,* **86,** (27), 50–52.

Plassman, B.L. and Breitner, J.C.S. (1996) Recent advances in the genetics of Alzheimer's disease and vascular dementia with emphasis on gene–environment interactions. *Journal of the American Geriatric Society.* **44,** 1242–1250.

Post, S.G. (1994) Genetics, ethics and Alzheimer's disease. *Journal of the American Geriatrics Society.* **42,** 782–786.

Spradley, J.P. (1979) *Participant Observation.* Holt Reinhart, New York.

Wallace, M. (1994) The sundown syndrome. *Geriatric Nursing,* May/June, 164–166.

Watson, R. (1997) Ethnomethodology and textual analysis. In: *Qualitative Research: Theory, Method and Practice,* (ed. D. Silverman), Sage Publications, London, pp. 80–98.

Wright, M. (1990) Reducing stress in carers. *The Carer,* **13,** 8–9.

7 CONCLUSIONS

Now that we have considered many of the aspects of the national picture of care for people with dementia and also seen how training to be self-directed in caring for this client group can be conducted, and the responses to such an approach, it is important to give some indication of how improvements can be made. The suggestions in this chapter are directly related to the contents of the book and I will try to indicate where these contents can be found, so that you may, if you wish, return to the pages on which the original issue was raised.

STAYING IN BUSINESS

On page 1 we discussed good principles, particularly as they relate to small businesses. The first of these, 'Determining the key factors for success in your business', is probably the most relevant here. Although it is well recognised that care for older people in the UK is inefficient in its funding and less than transparent in the amount and availability of resources (Sutherland, 1999, pp. xvii–xviii), some care organisations manage their business better than others. However, not being in control of your market (as this is mostly controlled by referral from social work) is a key factor that makes the private care sector different from most other businesses. Despite this, the key features of the care sector for older people, such as recruiting staff who, with training, will be motivated to provide good-quality care and remain with the organisation to become loyal employees, often determine the good organisation from the less good. Therefore those in management positions have an essential task to develop their staff and to encourage them to understand their role in the organisation and how they affect its functioning in a very direct way, in order to promote loyalty and good-quality care. The reputation of the organisation will depend on it.

So, managers need to have a vision of the goals of their organisation, be able to transmit these goals to their staff and encourage staff to take on the goals and to develop their role accordingly. As we discussed on page 21, carers often undertake their role because they enjoy the work anyway, so involving them in the organisation in every way makes good sense. This could include, as we saw on pages 25 and 26, developing the aims of the business with the staff (the business plan), reviewing the objectives (how it will work in practice, including the quality of life for those being cared for) and evaluating its effectiveness (looking at how the staff and the organisation as a whole have performed against the aims). Therefore being truly in touch with staff views will be vital.

Some organisations see the key to success not only in staff training but in following this with supervision, so that the implications of the training are realised in practice and any problems rectified. Vocational qualifications as a system also encourage this, despite their many other failings. The approach of training combined with supervision can also lead to a better co-ordinated workforce as well as one where the managers are closely involved in the day-to-day care. Provided it can be done in a sense of friendship and genuine concern for the carer as well as those being cared for, such a system need not appear oppressive. It could have the potential to lead to Levering's points (1994) a 'great place to work' that I have indicated on pages 27 and 28.

However, training does need to be based on the most up-to-date knowledge and this is where life-long learning comes into its own. What I have suggested here is that senior care staff be encouraged to develop these skills, so that they can not only train but can also supervise other staff to ensure a good quality of care along the lines of the organisation's goals. This will increase the motivation of the senior care staff so that they, in turn, will have more to contribute. For those with training budgets, it might be appropriate to release senior care staff occasionally for a few hours from work, so they can find and become familiar with appropriate material in relevant areas, rather than sending them on courses. This approach would also demonstrate the organisation's commitment to them as valued members of staff.

Let there be no doubt about it, there is no alternative to developing a way of working that incorporates educational principles. As the consultation paper *The Learning Age* (DCEE, 1998) shows, we are in an age where continual learning is essential.

STAFF TRAINING AND THE POTENTIAL FOR LIFE-LONG LEARNING: SOME GENERAL PRINCIPLES

In considering the potential for life-long learning in senior care staff in a number of different organisations, I have shown, on pages 32–39, the role the organisation needs to play. The organisation as a whole needs to be sufficiently encouraging and motivating to the individual in order for life-long learning to be a reality. Therefore, where the entire emphasis is on getting through the work, despite the abilities of individuals to be interested and willing to learn from the work, then the whole enterprise stifles individual interest. It may indeed consider interest in the work to be unnecessary. However, as we have seen throughout this book, the demands of those likely to refer older people for care (such as social workers) require that learning and keeping up to date are ongoing. So it seems, at worst, that there is little option to developing a system of life-long learning in care of people with dementia; at best, it could be a really exciting and rewarding prospect for everyone.

There are some general points that I would like to make about encouraging life-long learning in care of people with dementia, before we consider the organisations with which I worked.

- Senior staff need to give credit to employees who show an interest in their work to encourage them to want to discuss aspects of it with others. They should also provide a forum for this discussion to take place, for example at handover reports between the shifts. Employees should be encouraged to share their observations and suggestions with others in a system of mutual respect and support. Managers should allow these ideas (provided they are safe) to be tried and implemented by everyone so that the results can be evaluated in the discussion forums. Managers and senior care staff can facilitate this process so that everyone is encouraged to contribute.
- When recruiting staff, managers should bear in mind that improved levels of qualifications usually imply a more questioning approach to work. Provided questioning is accepted as part of the work, this raises the whole level of interest and gives everyone an opportunity to be involved.

- All staff should be helped to question their work and to encourage such an approach in others, particularly at times when staff are together, such as handover reports.

- As a result of questions being raised, staff need to be supported to try out new ideas (provided they are safe) under supervision to see what happens (evaluation) and to report back in discussion forums.

- Questioning can be very useful for the organisation when it is channelled into considering the conditions in which work and care are provided. Questioning can then be used to find ways to improve conditions for everyone.

- All staff should be encouraged to be responsible for their own education. Openly recognising each member of staff as having expertise in a specific area can help to develop such an approach. If the organisation is able to build up a small stock of books and journals in relevant areas, this might also help.

- A friendly and warm manner to staff as well as to those being cared for makes a world of difference to how everyone feels and the amount of effort they are willing to contribute.

These general principles are developed from the emphasis on life-long learning by Mezirow (1981) found on pages 36 and 38.

The issues that are discussed between staff and which form the way in which learning is promoted in the organisation are in line with the 'empowering' strategy that we considered on pages 50 and 51. It is empowering not only because care staff will have a very real say in how care is conducted and therefore in their own conditions of work but it will also be empowering for clients, because care staff often have closer relationships with clients than the senior staff or the managers. I have therefore assumed that the discussion between staff will be in the clients' best interests which will continue to raise the quality of care provided.

STAFF TRAINING AND THE POTENTIAL FOR LIFE-LONG LEARNING: THE EXPERIENCE OF THE ORGANISATIONS IN THE STUDY

As I have indicated throughout this book, the organisations with whom I worked have very different approaches to learning and showed a variety of responses to the relatively new idea of self-directed learning. However, they are by no means the only responses which could have been given, so I am not claiming that they are representative of every organisation involved in care for people with dementia. They are merely interesting examples.

If we relate the bullet points on pages 103–104 above to the organisations with whom I worked, we can see how they compare. I will develop this in the sequence in which the points arose in the previous chapters.

On page 67 we saw how, on the precourse questions, one of the participants indicated that she was highly likely to be self-directed in her learning already. However, she seemed to have little inclination to pass this on or to develop it in her staff. In such a situation, although one individual may pursue her own goals, she is not enabling anyone else. For the organisation as a whole to develop life-long learning in all its staff, most employees need to show a commitment and enthusiasm for the approach. A single individual practising it is unlikely to be able to make this change unless they make a very definite and sustained effort to change the organisation's culture and are able to take a number of other staff with them. To change an organisation's culture can be a very stressful business, as we saw on page 49, and maybe this individual was unwilling or did not have the confidence to do so or maybe she had tried and failed previously.

In organisation A (for their response see pages 75–81) there was a definite interest by carers in learning from work. However, they appeared to do this in isolation, as none of their diaries showed any of them making an impact on any of the other carers, whether senior or junior. It would seem fair to assume that, despite the manager saying that she came on the course in order to encourage the staff to pass on the information to those who did not attend, she was not able to do this. This organisation would be a very good example of where an attempt to encourage staff to share their observations of clients so that they might all learn from each other could have very positive results. If carers are helped to consider this as a useful activity, which is part of the work, then it could become a regular feature. However, once begun, it cannot be stifled and managers may fear losing control of the situation. Therefore it takes a great deal of courage for managers to foster this approach and they may need to be convinced that it is worth the effort. If it results in lower staff turnover, because staff feel that their interests and concerns are taken seriously, the effort will have been well worthwhile.

Therefore, from my experience, critical evaluation of one's work is to be applauded. However, it has little value to the client unless it is shared and accepted by everyone.

From the response to my input from organisation E (see pages 88–91) their need for knowledge from outside the organisation was evident. They also had a specific reason for wanting this knowledge and had thought carefully about why they wanted it and what they would use it for. However, although they said they benefited from outside stimulation, they appeared to be limited in finding resources for themselves; maybe a mentor or someone to 'bounce ideas off' was what they needed. They seemed to have limited confidence in how to find information so someone who could direct them to sources and show them how to make use of them would maybe help. Having the time to carry out such an activity is an issue that they may need to address.

Therefore, their response was nearer to self-directed learning than any of the other organisations but a few more steps needed to be taken for them to be fully launched.

Organisation C (for their response see pages 83–86) had one very keen senior carer who had been involved in education for a period of years. Her need for knowledge was evident and she was able to express her needs and evaluate the information received. However, she did not appear to appreciate that her colleague was experiencing considerable stress in the new organisation and needed more stability in her daily working, rather than a search for new knowledge. A slower pace was possibly needed for this senior carer to adjust. The same kind of difference in pace was seen in organisation G, where one senior carer had enormous energy and willingness to learn while the others were more pedestrian.

In the other organisations there was a need to consider how education could make a difference to their daily lives. Without this recognition it will be difficult for them to appreciate how questioning work, finding alternative answers, weighing them up and learning what works by trying different approaches can make a difference and can also improve the quality of care for people with dementia.

To finish, I would like to pay tribute to all the organisations with whom I worked and with whom I currently work. I realise that they are involved in a very difficult area and have continual problems in providing what they would ideally like to provide. There is no doubt in my mind that they all work enormously hard and have the clients' best interests at heart. However, I hope that what I have said here will help them to feel it is all worthwhile. I wish them all well.

REFERENCES

Department for Education and Employment (1998) *The Learning Age*. Cm 3790. The Stationery Office, London.

Levering, R. (1994) *A Great Place to Work*. Random House, New York.

Mezirow, J. (1981) A critical theory of adult learning and education. *Adult Education*, **32(1)**, 3–24.

Sutherland, S. (1999) *With Respect to Old Age: Long Term Care – Rights and Responsibilities*. A Report by the Royal Commission on Long Term Care. The Stationery Office, London.

APPENDIX 1
DIARY ENTRIES FROM ORGANISATION A IN THE FOLLOW-UP PERIOD

(The initials at the end of each entry are the carer's name)

AM

13.6.96
8am–6pm Today A's mood was very good. She responded well to anything that was said to her. Whilst toileting her she was very calm and did not get upset as she does normally. She has eaten well and has had plenty fluids.
IK

14.6.96
3pm–10pm A's mood fine and eating well. Sat in lounge. When going to bed very agitated when toileting her, very reluctant to sit on toilet even when bowels were moving. Reluctant to take clothes off although wanting to go to bed.
MC

15.6.96
A's mood fine, very relaxed and was laughing. Got her ready for bed, washed her and she even gave her teeth without any problems. Morning A in good mood, ate a good breakfast laughing and talking.
JC, EM

16.6.96
3pm–10pm A sitting in lounge very contented. A visit from her daughter C and her husband and youngest son. A very pleased to see them, especially

her grandson. She did not recognise them by name. A happy and changed and washed for bed with no problems.
MC

17.6.96
8am–6pm A was in a great mood. She wanted to get up this morning washed and dressed with no problems. Had breakfast in her room, drinking well and eating well. Have noted A's mood changes, when I put my hair up she never recognises me. When I had my hair down A was laughing and talking again.
JL

18.6.96
8am–6pm Today I helped her out of bed. Washed, dressed and sat her in her chair. She kept pointing to the picture of C. Very cheerful but tired. Brought A down for lunch. She ate everything on her plate. Only toileted her the once, due to circumstances, but she was dry.
IK

19.6.96
No entry

20.6.96
A is in great fettle today. Has eaten and drank well. She has been a delight to look after. I think her cheerfulness is due to a bowel movement, as when she is constipated, she is very tetchy.
IK

21.6.96
8am–6pm Had a long lie until 10.30am. Mood very changeable. When toileting her, found her to be wet twice. Has eaten and drank well. Have not noticed much change in A at all.
IK

21.6.96
3pm–10pm A very agitated when being put to bed. Very reluctant to allow me to wash her lower half. Refused to take her lower teeth out, went back 10 minutes later and still agitated but allowed me to remove teeth.

22.6.96
A was in a good mood today and she is a lot better when being toileted. A enjoyed having her tea in the lounge and the singsong.
AM

23.6.96
A was still in a good mood and joining in when we were dancing and singing in the lounge.
AM

24.6.96
A in very good form this morning. Enjoyed her porridge, drinking well, no problems.
ML

A was in a brilliant mood today, we gave her one of O's teddy's to see how she reacted and the reaction was great and A thought it was lovely.
MM

25.6.96
Was very bright and in a good mood. Is reacting well to the teddy she has been given.
EN

26.6.96
Had a sleep in the lounge before supper. Was in a good mood when assisted to get ready for bed.
EN

27.6.96
am A's mood was very cheerful despite the fact she was covered in faeces. A's mood seems to change when she has trouble with her bowels. Did not have any breakfast as she had a long lie, but ate a hearty lunch.
IK

pm A has been in an excellent mood all day. Eating and drinking well, laughing and joining in with all the care staff. When being assisted to get

ready for bed A's mood changed, and was not co-operative when getting undressed, would not allow me to take her teeth out, but managed to eventually. A in good spirits after getting into bed.
SS

28.6.96
am A was incontinent of faeces this morning, so therefore was not too enamoured about having a bath. Once A was washed and dressed, taken downstairs, she was fine. Eaten and drank well.
MW

29.6.96
am A in good form this am. Eating and drinking well. Still eating with her fingers laughing and pulling faces at staff.
AG

30.6.96
pm A very aggressive tonight did not want to get undressed.
AS

2.7.96
5pm–10pm A's mood good and talking a little while in the kitchen when having her meal. Very happy and settled down well when being prepared for bed. No problems giving me her teeth.
MC

3.7.96
8am–3pm A had a bath this morning upset when getting hair washed and weighed. Given her teddy which helped to calm her while I was drying her and her hair and this helped a lot.
MC

4.7.96
A went up the stairs all right, and got her ready for her bed, was all right until I went to take her teeth out. Was quite abusive, but eventually calmed down.
EM

5.7.96
A fine this evening, co-operative in undressing, slightly aggravated when asked to take her teeth out, and when assisted with personal hygiene.
SS

6.7.96
A in high spirits this am, fine when being washed and dressed, considering she had been incontinent of faeces. Eating and drinking well.
SS

Has been in a good mood all afternoon was laughing with care staff. Was not happy about having her teeth taken out and cleaned.
EN

7.7.96
A very tired when being put to bed and was very agitated. Tried giving her the teddy but this did not help. Was distressed when asking for teeth. Returned 10 minutes later and got teeth but not happy.
MC

8.7.96
5pm–10pm When putting A to bed tonight she was very aggressive with me also when trying to get her undressed she slapped my face and started to swear at me, once I got her over to her bed and she started to lie down she was fine.
AS

9.7.96
8am–2pm A not in a good mood this morning, shouting and swearing when put in the bath and also when drying and dressing her. Took her along to the hairdresser's room to have her hair done and seemed quite happy to sit with the rest of the ladies.
MM

12.7.96
A went to bed all right tonight, even managed to get her teeth without a problem.
EM

13.7.96
A ate well this evening, co-operated well, when being assisted to bed.
MM

14.7.96
A fine this morning, allowed me to wash and dress her without any problem. Ate and drank well.
MA

5pm–10pm A very happy sat with a soft toy, a bee. Undressed for bed without any difficulty and gave carer top teeth on her own. I slipped out the bottom teeth with very little trouble. A bit unhappy when applying cream to bottom.
MC

22.7.96
8am–5pm A is in a pleasant mood today, is fine until carer goes near her to toilet her or wash hands and face, but otherwise generally happy. Eating and drinking very well.
SS

25.7.96
5pm–10pm A is quite aggressive and abusive on taking her up the stairs and getting her ready for bed.
EM

26.7.96
5pm–10pm A was a little better tonight when getting ready for bed, but as soon as I went to take her teeth out she started getting abusive.
EM

27.7.96
5pm–10pm A was all right tonight going to her bed.
EM

28.7.96
5pm–10pm A in a very good mood when in the kitchen for meal in evening and ate well. When preparing for bed got a little aggressive. Gave her one of

her teddies and sat with her talking and playing with teddy until she was laughing again and then finished getting her ready for bed with no trouble.
MC

29.7.96
8am–6pm A was in a very good mood this morning. She laughed all the time while dressing. It wasn't until she came downstairs for lunch that her mood changed. Whilst having her lunch in the kitchen she is being tormented too much and this is upsetting her even more. It takes a while to calm her down. This cannot be good for A at all.
IM

5pm–10pm A is very agitated when going to bed tonight, when taking A's clothes off she started hitting at me and swearing quite a lot. I couldn't really get A calmed down so put her to bed as soon as possible. May this have something to do with the incident at lunchtime?
AS

31.7.96
A was in very good spirits before taking upstairs, carer was having a good time and laughing with her. A was fine until I was cleaning A's face, and personal hygiene use. A became abusive and calling names, waving her hands around. Once I got her teeth out A lay down and settled well.
LS

AC

5.7.96
5pm–10pm On getting A ready for bed she was very restless going back and forwards from the toilet to the door she did not want her clothes taken off because she was very cold, once ready for bed sat her in the lounge where she continued to get up and down asking for her sister put on some music for her and she seems to have settled down a bit.
AS

6.7.96
5pm–10pm Slept until 8.30am, had been up to the commode herself,

passed urine, got herself back to bed. Much more settled today than she was yesterday evening. But is still quite drowsy this am.
SS

6.7.96
Had to put A in bed early tonight as she was really very tired. And she was still sleeping when I left.
AS

7.7.96
When getting A into her nightclothes tonight she was getting quite annoyed because she keeps saying she is very unhappy, so one of the carers played the piano for her but she was still very restless.
AS

8.7.96
2pm–10pm A has been restless all afternoon, unable to settle for any length of time. A was incontinent of urine twice – at 3pm and 6pm. A was observed to be overfilling her mouth at teatime, almost greedy.
JE

9.7.96
A in quite a good mood and was left longer after dinner, mood turned when trying to get A undressed, no matter how much talking and coaxing was given A was unco-operative especially when I tried to get her teeth out. Once bathed and dressed for bed A flaked out.
AS

12.7.96
Has been settled today. She had a visit from R this afternoon. Has been settled the rest of the evening.
EN

13.7.96
A was fine all day today, very chatty, pleasantly confused.
SS

14.7.96
Has been wandering a lot tonight. Asking for her sister and asking where she stayed.
EN

16.7.96
A woke up at 8.45 and seemed more settled, was shown a lot of soft toys to ask if she would like one but did not want one. A more alert today.
MC

20.7.96
A has been asking for her sister all morning and wanting to go home.

At approx. 3pm A had wandered out the front door and fell, thus cutting her head on the wall. Was taken to (local hospital) straight away, but not returning until 9pm.

22.7.96
8am–5pm A was up and dressed by 8am this morning. She was her usual chatty self, not sleeping too much today and is not wandering at all. A was joining in with activities in the lounge this afternoon with other residents. Eating + drinking well.
SS

25.7.96
A is very restless tonight, calling out and shouting for help.
LH

26.7.96
Is more settled tonight and has been in a good frame of mind. Is still sleeping on and off.
EN

27.7.96
Eating and drinking well, not wandering so much, but still being repetitive saying nurse, nurse, help me, help me!
SS

28.7.96
A was all right at tea-time, but from 6 o'clock onwards was starting to wander again and asking for a nurse to help her repeatedly.
EM

29.7.96
A was great tonight down in lounge all night and watched television.
AS

31.7.96
A has been very restless all night is not settling very well in lounge. She is asking about her family a lot tonight. Wanting to go home.
AS

5.8.96
A was restless again tonight, took her up to her bed at 9.45pm, as she had wet herself and had to be changed into clean nightware.
EM

APPENDIX 2
PRE-COURSE INFORMATION

What is your experience of people with dementia?

What did you feel like looking after these people with dementia?

Why did you come on the course?

What do you hope to be able to do at the end of the course that you could not do before it?